Paradise Health

A Feasting and Fasting Guide to
Optimal Health through Detoxification

Volume 1

KHEPRA ANU

Khepra's Raw Food Juice Bar

402 H St NE

Washington, DC 20002

Phone: 202.803.2063

E-mail: khepra@chefkhepra.com
www.kheprasrawfoodjuicebar.com

Edited by: Carol Solon
             Beverly Green
Layout Design by Aza Nedhari
Cover Design by Mark L. Milligan II

DISCLAIMER

The techniques and advice described in this book represent the opinions of the author, based on his experience. The author expressly disclaims any responsibility for any liability, loss or risk, personal or otherwise, which is incurred as a result of using any of the techniques, recipes or recommendations suggested herein. If in any doubt or, if requiring medical advice, please contact the appropriate health professional.

This book is dedicated with all my love

to my beloved son, Khemra As Anu, who left

us at six months of age and entered eternal

Paradise.

TABLE OF CONTENTS

INTRODUCTION

Fasting and feasting properly as a continual way of life is the only way to live better, more vibrantly, and to truly avoid age-related infirmities. Fasting is one extreme and Feasting is the other, each equally important, and when done systematically and scientifically, form a harmonious dance of yin and yang, soft and hard, fast and slow. Unfortunately for most of us, living in a land that reveres consumption, fasting only occurs when one is either asleep or ill. Little do we realize that both sleep and illness are programmed into the body's cycle, so that at a minimum, we can allow the digestive and other body systems to rest! With our having a constant consumer mindset, we might eat around the clock! This would put the body into a crisis that would force illness, which then would shut down the appetite but, nevertheless, allow the body a well-deserved and healing rest. For optimal health, voluntary fasts are as necessary and as important as any other health supplement, practice, program, or regimen. If you are not regularly fasting as a lifestyle practice, then you haven't experienced true paradise health.

Living according to Nature's Laws is the next New Age phenomenon on the horizon in which select ideas and philosophies will be presented for optimal living. Violation of our natural diet alone has damaged our health and supports dogmatic "sickcare" industries that serve to profit from our chronic disease and, eventually, our premature demise. The study of Nature, including the cosmos, gives us clear indications not only as to what we should eat, but how much, and the optimal times of day in which to eat. The information presented in this body of work can serve as a model to follow, along with the cycles of Nature that occur systematically throughout every season. By understanding and incorporating these philosophies into our lives, we can begin our journey towards realizing the human potential of true health and happiness for ourselves, our families, and communities.

When we examine self-development from the standpoint of mind, body, and spirit, we can only do so much without food either being the foundation or a primary pillar in that foundation of growth and development. The old maxim, "You are what you eat" will always be true. We are only fooling ourselves by reaching a level of personal mastery in an area in which we have devoted decades of blood, sweat and tears. We don't consider the fuel that we run on daily as not being of primary importance. Our spiritual body existed before we came into our physical body. Yet, we must ask the question, "How can we consider ourselves spiritually, mentally, or emotionally adept when our physical bodies are not in perfect working order?"

Our physical temple houses our spirit or ethereal body. If our house is dirty, everything else is in chaos. When we have physical pain or our eyes and teeth are in a steady state of decay, or we are taking over-the-counter medications, we are simply not in divine spiritual, mental and emotional alignment. Our bodies are breaking down prematurely, primarily from improper food choices.

It is vitally important to realize that regarding food and the health of our bodies, there are only two types of food: food that creates mucus and food that is mucus-less or mucus-free, as the great Professor Arnold Ehret pointed out in his works over a century ago. The only foods that are mucus-free in the body are fruits and green leafy vegetables. Everything else is mucus-forming food, including nuts and seeds. (That is why nuts and seeds should usually be soaked before eating in order to release enzyme inhibitors, and then should be eaten in moderation.) We have come to realize that fruits and vegetables should comprise the largest part of our diet. Eating a basically fruitarian diet should be everyone's goal to living a healthy long-lasting life, free of disease. In addition to proper diet/proper feasting, fasting becomes an integral part of the lifestyle. When we fast, we "quicken" the healing process. I believe this is part of the reason why it is called a "fast." No matter what the reason is why you are fasting, everything will happen "faster" than if you were eating day in and day out. With a proper mucus-free feasting regimen along with periodic fasting, the fasting will allow the body to heal more quickly than if fasting was not a part of the regimen.

Over the years during which I have been practicing a live food vegan diet, I have researched, experimented and studied a wide array of philosophies that exist even within the raw food movement. Most "experts" (i.e., leaders, authors, authorities) agree that the raw food diet primarily consists of fresh fruits, vegetables, nuts and seeds and sprouted grains. The difference basically lies with the percentage of intake necessary in the four groups of foods.

There also are subgroups within the primary groups. Considering fruits as a primary group example, there are high water content sweet fruits and denser fatty fruits. To use these foods scientifically for the purpose of healing oneself, it becomes very important to understand when and how to apply these two different fruit subgroups, which are botanically similar. My aim is to simplify this mass of information and make it suitable and purposeful for this guide. When I do research or meditate on the "perfect" healing system and diet, the answer always comes back to balance. I will present what I believe to be a balanced healing and diet program that will put us on the path to paradise health.

The most important realization that I have had based on my experiences and the experiences of others is that fasting is a life-long practice. Most people who have undergone a voluntary fast at least once in their lifetime may approach fasting as something they do at least annually or once in a blue moon. There is nothing wrong with that approach; however, anyone who has had the experience of fasting multiple times can tell you that, subsequent to each fast, he/she feels closer to savoring the vitality of his/her own potential. This is the key when considering that after each fast, we become "cleaner" and can catch glimpses of our divine path.

The aim of this guide serves multiple purposes. First, this guide represents my formula for the attainment of perfect health or what I like to call Paradise Health. Most of the juices and water that is taken in during this designed detox are from foods that are found in Paradise. I believe that by drinking coconut water or the nectar of a sugar cane stalk, you are ingesting paradise created by the grand master chef, Mother Nature. You slowly become Paradise because you are what you eat. By this idea alone, my hope is that you will be inspired to do the best you can do. One of my maxims is: "It's not where you are at, it's where you are headed." We are all headed in one direction or another. Our daily habits determine in which direction we are headed. Ask yourself this question, "With my daily diet and lifestyle, am I creating paradise health or am I headed for disease, pain, suffering, and premature death?" The human spirit always wants to keep growing and improving and challenging itself to be better.

The second purpose of this guide is to help you understand the true nature of disease, as well as the nature of vitality. Understanding that if food is primary and integral to our vitality, then any healing system that doesn't deal with food as a foundation is—in my opinion—at best, misleading and false.

The third aim of this guide is to touch on areas of our lives at the times when the discipline of proper feasting and fasting can make all the difference. Whatever your choice might be for improving your physical temple; let it be worthwhile for you. It could be that you are sick and tired of being sick and tired. You could be motivated to cure yourself of an "incurable" disease. Or, you would like to reverse the aging process and look more youthful, sexy, and attractive. These and many other reasons are all valid for making proper fasting and feasting a foundation of our lifestyles. I passionately feel that we owe paradise health to ourselves, because our bodies are the only thing we truly own in this physical reality in which we live. Why not strive to get a glimpse of how good you can really look and feel?

The last aim of this guide is to introduce a scientific system of fasting that is not only fun but, I personally feel, the best way to cleanse as

Mother Nature herself intended for every human being. There is comprehensive information here to help you succeed on your detox program. Enjoy this manual and also be inspired to see and begin a new chapter of your life!

FASTING AND FEASTING

I like to put the words feasting and fasting together because one balances the other, like yin and yang. I think that most of us can say that we've spent all of our lives voluntarily feasting a lot more than voluntarily fasting. This fact wouldn't be so bad if our primary foods were uncultivated, wild, organic fruits, and vegetables. Since that is not the case, as a people we are sorely out of balance. Now, for us as a greater community to realize our human potential, we must systematically and scientifically fast on a regular basis to take control of our health and well-being.

Feasting in today's culture has become an addiction that is no different from any other addiction that plagues humanity today. I would argue that it is by far the worst and most deadly addiction, because a large part of our society is so accepting of it. Most, if not all, cigarette smokers, especially given the recent court cases over the years and from the good work of non-profit organizations, know that their addictive habit is not a good one. It is difficult for smokers to find areas, other than outside their office buildings or at their local bars, to smoke freely without catching flack about spreading their toxic second-hand smoke. However, who frowns upon those enjoying a hamburger or pizza for lunch, a stack of pancakes with coffee for breakfast, a low-fat Subway sandwich, or even the gluten or tofu meat imitations at their local vegan restaurants? You can argue which one is "healthier" than another, but all of them are addictive and will result in a breakdown of our priceless body temple. It is only when we make a habit of scientific fasting, along with a proper feasting regimen in our lives, that we can then understand what is truly addictive to our palate.

We must first and foremost be thankful for the expansion in the greater consciousness of humanity for the demand of organic foods. This has created better health for ourselves, families, and communities and has been a more sustainable form of agribusiness for the Earth, our only home.

However, we cannot rest on these laurels. You can walk into a Whole Foods Market and mistakenly purchase a genetically-modified apple when you thought you were buying an organic one. Whole Foods, a market that prides itself as being the largest retailer of organic produce, also sells its fair share of pesticide-ridden conventional produce and genetically-modified laboratory-created freak food. Our food has been refined to a level where our choices largely rely upon what is good for agribusiness.

The feasting and fasting regimen starts with an understanding of nature's food groups. When taking on a week-long fast, especially for the first time, it is essential to have a balance between your intake of the three dominant elements present in your juices (when fasting) and then in your food (when feasting). There are a few subcategories within the big three but, for the purpose of simplicity, we will discuss the main three.

The first group is sugar dominant foods, which consist mostly of our juicy wet fruits. It is worth mentioning that non-sweet fruits, such as cucumber and tomato, are a subcategory of the first group. The second is our bitter or protein dominant foods, which is composed of the green leafy vegetable family. The third is the oil or fat dominant group, which contains all our nuts, seeds, and fruits, such as olives, avocados, and durian, just to name a few. When we are feasting, all three dominant groups are included in food preparation and should create a balance. Different nutritional authorities in the raw food community vary greatly in their opinion as to the ideal ratio for human consumption among the three food categories.

For the purposes of this guide and because most of us are toxic from lifelong abuse, fasting rather than feasting is emphasized. For the best detox, juices blended or extracted from sweet water dominant fruits are our primary intake. This gives our body an opportunity to consume fat reserves in our tissues and; therefore, allows us to lose weight. Most toxins are stored in fat reserves as well. However, when doing other flushes, such as the liver flush, oils in the form of olive oil, hemp or flax oil are effective in driving out cholesterol residues that choke the liver and could ultimately create a gallstone problem. Green juices are always useful, especially when mineral deficiencies are present and when a heavy metal detoxification is needed.

Most people are interested in losing weight when undertaking a detoxification program. On average, most participants will lose 5-10 lbs a week of detoxification. However, I have had a number of people interested in not losing too much weight during a fast. These same people are usually interested in gaining weight because they feel that they are underweight, especially women. On the other hand, women of African descent have an added pressure due to the fact that it has become an African aesthetic for women to have some meat on their bones, or to be affectionately called "thick." I feel that, whether seeking to lose or gain weight, these are legitimate concerns, and we must aspire to be healthier, cleaner, and more vibrant. Our first objective has to be a clean and healthy inside. Without that as the foundation, whether our systems break down more seriously by disease, whether the breakdown is more cosmetic, such as wrinkles, gray or balding hair, or whether there is a loss of energy and vitality, it is tragic and could be avoided.

WEIGHT LOSS

Obesity is a disease. A simple remedy for the cure of being overweight combines a proper diet and lifestyle. However, hindering the success of weight loss for most people is the hype of buying convenient processed foods and the overindulgence of cooked starchy foods; it's of epidemic proportions. I characterize the remedy as simple, but it is not. Starchy foods include rice, bread, pasta, grains, beans, legumes and root vegetables, such as potatoes, yams, and yucca.

Cooked or processed foods require a high amount of heat in order to make these foods more digestible by increasing the water content. For example, pasta or rice needs to be boiled in water so that it can be soft enough to chew. From a nutritional standpoint, we understand that starchy foods are a carbohydrate or sugar; they are in a complex form. Hence, we have the term complex carbohydrate. Simple carbohydrates or simple sugars are what we find naturally in fresh fruits; these sugars are in perfect balance with the amount of water and fiber present and, therefore, easy for the body to process and digest. For complex carbohydrates, the complexity of the sugar makes it very difficult for these foods to be broken down in the body. Because these foods are not suitable for the human body to digest, and they are very high in sugar, we always combine starches with protein or fat dominant foods. Thus, the primary reason for overweight human bodies is the improper food combination of proteins and starch.

The protein-starch combination is presumably the most addictive food combination ever created. Any time we eat a meal, there is almost always a starch combined with protein. Let's list some examples: baked potato with butter or cheese, rice with butter or gravy and bread with meat, tuna and/or cheese. We get that false-sense-of-comfort feeling of fullness and satisfaction. The worst part of the protein-starch combination is that the body is unable to digest protein and starch simultaneously. Nothing gets digested efficiently. The food sours and ferments, leading to intestinal gas. The body then becomes a refinery by transforming the starch into alcohol. The effect of the alcohol produced in the body from cooked starch, ill-combined with protein/fat, is highly addictive. The key is to avoid or at least begin to wean oneself off of starch.

16

Fat and oil in food is NOT the issue. Avocados, olives, nuts, seeds, coconut jelly, durian, jackfruit, and all natural sources of fat and protein will NOT make you fat. An interesting point is that the removal of starch from the diet is the only reason why people participating in the Atkins diet are able to lose weight. With the Atkins diet, you can eat everything except starch, including dairy and meat. Any form of protein is allowable just as long as the starch is avoided.

The best way to wean off starch is to focus on dark green leafy vegetables, such as kale, spinach, red leaf, green leaf and romaine lettuces and chard, mustard and collard greens. If you are not a "salad" person, work to become one. It does not matter what your blood type is or whether you are a fast or slow metabolizer. It is vital to eat your greens raw. If you need to, steam them lightly; however, with your delectable homemade dressings (see recipe section for ideas), once you add your extra virgin olive oil and other ingredients, the greens begin to break down almost immediately without the use of heat. It is criminal what cooks do to greens by slowly cooking the LIFE out of them. When you add the smooth olive oil, some kale greens, for example, will shine with that vibrant beautiful green color reminding you that it was the sun's energy responsible for bringing this nutritious and delicious green to your salad bowl.

It is also worth mentioning that the primary reason we lose our teeth is because we are not exercising them properly by chewing the foods that will naturally strengthen and nourish them. As a daily practice, it is EXCELLENT to chew a mouthful of green leafy vegetables with nothing added. This will revitalize your teeth, gums, and jaw to the point where you may never need to see a dentist!

Feasting for Weight Loss Daily Regimen

Pre-Breakfast (5 a.m. - 7 a.m.)

32-64 oz. Coconut water or distilled water with fresh lemon/lime

Breakfast – Meal 1 (8 a.m. – 10 a.m.)

1–3 lbs. High water content sugar fruit (melons, citrus, sub-acid)

Lunch – Meal 2 (12 noon – 2 p.m.)

Big green salad with homemade dressing and vegetable fruits

Snack – Meal 3 (4 p.m. – 5 p.m.)

Fresh celery sticks with raw almond butter or handful of soaked nuts or seeds

Dinner – Meal 4 (7 p.m. – 8 p.m.)

Vegetable protein source with green salad with homemade dressing and vegetable fruits

This may seem like a lot of food for one day, but the key to weight loss is food intake. Again, what will make it possible for your body to demand this amount of intake is to be very active. Therefore, in addition to a yoga/meditation practice, add in another more active form of movement, such as running, weight lifting, calisthenics, or dance.

WEIGHT GAIN

As a veteran faster and raw foodist, many people come to me, especially women, about their weight and their desire to either gain or keep the weight that they have. As seekers of health, the biggest sign of health is how we appear, how we look. No matter if we are presently slim or grossly overweight, the first day we begin to fast, weight loss will begin almost immediately. For the 7-day Khepra Juice Detox regimen, people lose on average 5-10 lbs per week. The overweight person is immediately pleased with the results. However, the slender individual who does not want to shed too many pounds now is caught between not wanting to lose too much weight and aspiring to be healthy through fasting.

While evolving into the beings of perfection that is our birthright, you may feel worse before you feel better. You will have to lose weight or lose the garbage before you can build a healthy sound body temple. You will have to go through a trial period in which you may look emaciated. However, it is at that point when your body has eliminated most of the waste in your lymph system that it is ready to build a healthy new foundation. This process can last on average about six months. With consistent periodic fasting, it can be much sooner.

What is the regimen to follow in order to gain healthy weight by eating primarily fruits, vegetables, nuts, seeds, and spouted grains? The answer is simple: eat high water sugar fruits for breakfast; eat a big salad using spinach, kale, or collard greens for lunch and repeat for dinner. With your greens, it is very important to include healthy oils or fats, such as avocados and/or olives, soaked seeds, such as pumpkin, sunflower, or hemp. (Hemp seeds are usually sold fresh, so they don't have to be soaked.) Seeds are superior to nuts, so use seeds more often than nuts for your healthy fats. In addition to those 3 meals, you would need to do at least 2 green smoothies per day in between breakfast and lunch, lunch and dinner, or after dinner. The exact schedule would depend on your workout routine. You will need to work out at least 3-4 times per week to stimulate your digestion, since you will be bringing in lots of nutrition with 5+ meals per day, every day. For example, if you prefer to work out in the mornings, you would do better to have your first smoothie after breakfast. Your second smoothie can be either after lunch or after dinner. If you work out in the early evenings, then you would do better to have a green smoothie after dinner. A suggested workout would be power yoga or an active yoga routine that strengthens muscle mass, but also keeps your body flexible and limber. For green smoothie recipes for weight gain, see recipe section in the Appendix.

Give this dietary regimen at least 90 consecutive days for sustained results. It may have to become your dietary lifestyle long after 90 days in order to keep the healthy weight that you have gained, and studies have shown that it takes 90 consecutive days for a routine to become a part of our nature. In addition, remember that the green smoothies are liquid meals, so they need to be spaced accordingly between your solid meals.

The last thing that is important to understand is that in order to put on healthy weight doing raw fruits and vegetables, you will have to more than likely lose weight before you gain the weight that you desire. This happens anyway when taking on the raw diet. Your body will go into a level of detoxification where the body will cleanse and lose the garbage that has been stored. The intelligence of the body will not allow it to build on a faulty foundation. On average, it takes between 3-6 months for most people to first lose the garbage and then begin to build the body. Thereafter, the body will start to build and settle at its natural weight. If more weight gain is desired beyond your natural weight, then it is important to follow the regimen stated below.

Feasting for Weight Gain Daily Regimen

Pre-Breakfast (5 a.m. – 7 a.m.)
32-64 oz. Coconut Water or distilled water with fresh lemon/lime

Breakfast – Meal 1 (8 a.m. -10 a.m.)
1–3 lbs High water content sugar fruit (melons, citrus, sub-acid)

Pre-Lunch -- Meal 2 (10 a.m. -11 a.m.)
Green smoothie (Blend 1 lb of greens with 2 cups of water; add fruit, nuts, avocado, and sweetener)

Lunch – Meal 3 (12 noon – 2 p.m.)
Big green salad with homemade dressing and vegetable fruits

Pre-Dinner -- Meal 4 (4 p.m. - 5 p.m.)
Green smoothie (Blend 1 lb. of greens with 2 cups of water; add fruit, nuts, avocado, and sweetener)

Dinner – Meal 5 (7 p.m. – 8 p.m.)
Big green salad with homemade dressing and vegetable fruits

This may seem like a lot of food for one day, but like weight loss, the key to weight gain is food intake. Again, what will make it possible for your body to demand this amount of intake is to be very active. In addition to a yoga/meditation practice, add in another more active form of movement like running, weight lifting, calisthenics or dance.

THE BUSINESS OF WATER

Water, with its great importance in sustaining life, has to be addressed, as it relates to our feasting and fasting regimen for higher health. There is a lot of miseducation and misinformation. What is important is that we are clear with its role in attaining greater vitality. Most of us believe that "all water is created equal," that we can pick up any spring or purified water from our local supermarket, drink at least 8 glasses a day and affect positive change in our bodies. What is worse is when we believe that we are doing our bodies a favor by drinking mineral rich or "hard" water. Think about what happens when mineral rich hard water is put in our iron to press clothes. Over time, you will see the residue that ultimately damages the iron. When we use distilled water, no residue forms. The mineral rich residue also is present in our shower heads. Similarly, those mineral residues are present in our bodies, in our joints, organs and cells. When we examine the water that Mother Nature produces for us, the water is usually in a distilled living form; it is "soft" water. Coconut water and water in all fruits and vegetables are all in a distilled living soft form. Rain water is another form of drinking water that in the right clean environment is distilled by the environment.

Coconut water is the most optimal form of living water. In analyzing the composition and mineral content of coconut water in comparison to drinking water, coconut proves to be superior in every respect for the following reasons: Minerals present in coconut water are organic minerals, whereas minerals found in tap water, spring water, salt water, vitamins, multi-vitamins, and mineral supplements are in an inorganic form. Organic minerals are living substances usable by the body. Inorganic minerals are dead and not usable by the body. Furthermore, what is not passed out through the urine can settle in different parts of the body, usually the joints. On the other hand, coconut water has the capability to nourish the body at the cellular level; the needed minerals are distilled and completely usable, even simultaneously removing from the joints, the blood, and other vital organs the inorganic minerals that plague the system.

If you cannot purchase coconut water, I suggest purchasing a water distiller and adding lemon and lime to your regular drinking water.

Lemons and limes are first-class mucus dissolvers and, with the mechanically created distilled water, you are essentially revitalizing the water.

Coconut water is whole and living water; you can live off coconut water and thrive as a human being. Coconut water is probably the only water that will cleanse every organ, every cell and all the blood throughout the body. The Sanskrit term for coconut translates into "all that is required to live." It is naturally designed to rid the body of mucus, inorganic mineral deposits, parasites and worms, and any other decomposed matter that may be present in the body. It is amazing to know that nature's water is equipped to do it all and that it TASTES GOOD! The moisture content will, over time, remove the mucoid plaque lining in your colon. Because it is also nourishing the body with vitamins, minerals, and electrolytes, you will have natural energy throughout your day. You will become a new you with the gift of Mother Nature, by taking in the best water as nature intended.

Fresh squeezed orange juice (OJ) will provide similar benefits. It is recommended that for every 10 oranges juiced, add the juice of one lime; or more lime if you love its sour flavor as I do. For the beginning faster, the duration of this part of the regime should last at least 3 days. For the more experienced faster, the coconut water/fresh OJ regimen can last much longer, depending on the level of "cleanliness" of your internal body. Another option in a sample 3-day period is to begin with OJ and coconut water, then do coconut water alone for day 2, and on the 3rd day, repeat the OJ and coconut water. This is an example of fasting scientifically, by allowing the body to gently adjust from food to lighter juices, then gradually completing the fast the same way you began, so that when you are finally ready to break your fast, you have complete control of your appetite.

COCONUT WATER - NATURE'S MASTER CLEANSER

Coconut water comes from the green water coconuts that grow in the tropical climate regions of the world. Coconut water was designed by Mother Nature herself to completely nourish and cleanse the temple of the human body. The water navigates its way from the ocean and minerals of the earth and travels through a perfect distillation process, moving upward through the long coconut palm tree, where it is collected and maintained in a pressurized green shell; the shell can sometimes appear yellow or orange, depending on the variety. Mother Nature has produced a perfect living water that vitalizes us, and once discovered, makes the transition back to commercial bottled water difficult. Coconut water will cleanse and nourish without the addition of any herbs, spices, or other additives. Given these, and many other innumerable qualities, water from the coconut is the Real Master Cleanser.

Before we continue with how and why the coconut is the Queen Mother of all foods and cleanses, let us look at what most people have come to know as the "Master Cleanse," or the Lemonade Diet. Stanley Burroughs created the lemonade recipe in 1941, and this cleansing recipe has been recently made popular by Peter Glickman. Many people, including celebrities, have undergone the lemonade diet with great results; this is a fantastic thing, as it shows that people are taking more responsibility for their health in this age of information and technology. People have a greater consciousness of diet when they see a direct correlation to their health.

The lemonade fast consists of water, fresh lemon juice, cayenne pepper, and maple syrup. What often is suggested for this particular fast is that a salt water flush and laxative tea also be included. If anyone is interested in doing this particular fast, I would make the following suggestions:

Use distilled water; to my knowledge, the recipe does not call for a specific type of water over another. However, all natural drinking water is distilled, or "soft" water. Coconut water is a soft distilled water, as is the water contained in all fruits and vegetables. You can either buy distilled water by the gallon or invest in a distiller.

Use coconut nectar rather than maple syrup or avoid sugar all together. Coconut nectar is a diabetic-safe sweetener that comes from the coconut flower bud. Unlike sugar, coconut nectar has a low-glycemic index, meaning it does not cause a sharp rise in blood sugar. Coconut nectar is a relatively new sweetener on the market. It has gone through very little processing and is one of the best sweeteners any health-conscious person should have available for juices, smoothies, desserts and dressings. What makes coconut nectar special is that it is processed from coconut blooms and almost entirely composed of inulin, a carbohydrate which can be beneficial to feeding the good bacteria in the large intestine. Agave has come under scrutiny given its high fructose content, some claiming that it is no better than high fructose corn syrup. Maple syrup is highly refined. Syrup from trees in its natural state is very bitter and, in order for the syrup to become sweet, it has to undergo multiple processes of boiling and refining. Coconut nectar, according to the latest research, is the superior alternative. However, my take is that a sweetener is a sweetener, regardless of the source or the processing, meaning that no additionally processed sugar is probably your best option.

Instead of cayenne pepper, practice yoga daily; The purpose of cayenne pepper is to stimulate blood flow. Cayenne pepper causes irritation in both the digestive lining and throughout the digestive system. By establishing a daily yoga practice, you will allow your blood and lymphatic system to move out the unnecessary toxins that are creating a blockage within the system. Yoga also will do much more in the way of exercise and healing the body, by allowing the body to become better aligned and more relaxed. If you are physically challenged or have an injury and find that yoga is not the best option, there are other forms of exercise that may be better suited for you. Walking, fire breathing, or doing whatever exercise is in sync with your body is recommended.

If you find it necessary to "spice" up your juice, I would strongly suggest using fresh jalapeño, habanero, or cayenne peppers. With dried cayenne pepper flakes, the drying process has made this an imbalanced food. Fresh peppers have the perfect balance of fiber, water, oil and heat, not to mention, the life force of the pepper is still intact.   With the dried pepper flakes, you have just heat and nothing else.   As a chef with years of experience making raw dishes, it is also extremely important to consider using fresh hot peppers over dried cayenne pepper flakes when looking to add fire to your dishes.

The so-called "master cleanser" or lemonade diet recommends implementing a salt and herbal tea regimen to assist in flushing the bowels.   The salt water and herbal tea, such as Smooth Move, stimulate your bowels to eliminate waste from your body.   However, the combination of herbs and salt water shocks the body through stimulation, rather than allowing the body the freedom to work the waste out of the body by its own power.   My thought is that, if the lemonade recipe is the master cleanser, why are salt and herbal laxative teas needed?   Drinking coconut water alone is sufficient for adequate nourishing and cleansing.   You can drink coconut water solely for months at a time and thrive.   Herbal teas and salt water do not measure up to the completeness of fresh coconut water.   Coconut water is a healing water, a drinking water, and a fasting water; it is the real master cleanser.

COCONUT WATER - A POTASSIUM POWERHOUSE

A few years ago, one of my detox clients, a man in his 60s, had undergone a series of coconut water fasts. He felt good enough to stop taking his medications for hypertension and diabetes. He was so 'gung-ho' about his health and vitality, but that wasn't enough for his mental well-being, he needed reassurance from his regular doctor. What he really longed for was to prove to a medically-trained doctor that what he was doing with fasting and his lifestyle was superior to drugs and medications. However, after having blood work done, the doctor saw that the patient's potassium levels were "through the roof." The doctor proceeded to give him injections to bring the blood potassium level down. The doctor scared my client into believing that a high potassium level is unhealthy and not normal. This led me to question whether we can overdose on potassium. Can we drink too much coconut water? Can we use coconut water as a replacement for spring or pure water? These were questions I had for years. When the role of potassium in the body is understood, then we are able to have the answers to these questions.

First, what does potassium do in the body? High levels of potassium in the body allow for muscle strength, high energy, quick reflexes, smooth digestion, high mental function, and joint and bone health. If you eat the Standard American Diet (SAD), then you are definitely deficient in potassium. Low potassium levels can lead to diabetes, hypertension, heart disease, and digestive issues, such as constipation, irritable bowel syndrome, heartburn, and hemorrhoids.

We also have to compare the ratio of potassium to sodium. For optimal health, there has to be an ideal balance of potassium to sodium. Our bodies should contain twice as much potassium as sodium. The majority of the foods we eat should contain much more potassium than sodium. Comparing the composition of most fruits, vegetables, nuts and seeds, we see that there is a large ratio of potassium to sodium content. A medium-sized banana, for example, has approximately 400 mg of potassium to 1 mg of sodium. An avocado has approximately 700 mg of potassium to 10 mg of sodium. Coconut water's sodium content can vary, depending on whether the coconut was grown near salt water shorelines or inland, where it pulls from salt-free rivers and streams. As a coconut connoisseur, I believe that the coconuts grown near salt water are the best and tastiest.

Salt water coconuts have an approximate ratio of 600 mg of potassium to 250 mg of sodium, whereas inland coconut water has a ratio of 450 mg of potassium to 25 mg of sodium. In contrast, processed foods have a much higher sodium content in relation to potassium. Cooked starches, which are the worst foodstuffs that we can eat, are naturally higher in sodium than potassium. Bagels have approximately 250 mg of sodium to only 40 mg of potassium. Wheat bread has approximately 130 mg of sodium to only 40 mg of potassium. Animal flesh and dairy products also have 5 to 10 times more sodium than potassium content. When potassium's role in the body is understood, it is a potassium deficiency that generally leads to high blood pressure rather than a sodium overdose. A diet high in potassium will balance a high intake of salt and not cause high blood pressure. Patients suffering from hypertension need to rebalance their potassium:sodium intake; that alone will balance the heart and allow for better blood flow. Potassium and sodium are electricity—or electrolytes—that allows for electrical impulses to occur throughout the body. When the ratio is balanced by eating mostly fresh fruits, vegetables, nut, and coconut water, our body responds by moving, thinking and living more efficiently and effectively.

I have been drinking coconut water as my primary water for at least 8 years. It has become very difficult, if not impossible, to return to "regular" water as my primary water source. Some authorities advise against replacing regular water with coconut water. However, coconut water hydrates the body better than pure water, because of the electrolytes. Coconut water has life, whereas spring water is inert. Coconut water flushes the colon and all the digestive organs, in addition to the kidneys, whereas spring water only flushes the kidneys. I will continue to drink coconut water, and I am willing to be the poster child guinea pig for putting coconut water as a primary water to the test. In addition to high potassium levels that coconut water contains, coconut water has the richest, highest levels of the anti-aging growth hormone, cytokinin. Cytokinins have been found to promote tissue growth, naturally thin the blood, kill cancer cells, promote elasticity and strength in the skin and stimulate strong hair growth.

Many juice enthusiasts are concerned about the "freshness" of juices. It is common knowledge that most fruits and vegetables lose freshness and enzymes immediately after blending or juicing. By using coconut water as a base for juice recipes, the freshness of juice need not be a concern because of the endosperm content of coconut water. Along scientific lines, seeds contain endosperm, which is the lifeblood of nourishment that allows a plant to mature from a seed into a fruit. Endosperm in seeds is a starchy, nutrient-dense substance. Coconuts, as seeds, contain liquid endosperm. The liquid endosperm of the coconut is coconut water! If the coconut remains unopened, the water will serve as the lifeblood of a future coconut palm.

Coconuts are the only food on the planet that has this phenomenal duality of seed and water. Given the nutritional characteristics of coconut water, coconuts do not lose their "freshness" once they are picked from the tree. In fact, the anti-aging hormones become more potent. Therefore, by using fresh coconut water in all of my juice recipes, loss of nutritional integrity is not a concern for the juices that I prepare for myself and my clientele.

THE FOUNTAIN OF YOUTH

I have come across a number of beliefs, philosophies, and practices that contribute to the notion of the eternal fountain of youth. Can we live eternally? Would we even want to? If you have yet to ask yourself these questions, fasting with regularity will most assuredly aid in the quest for longevity.

Most people desire to look youthful and stay healthy for a variety of reasons. It is our birthright to be the best, look the best and accomplish all we are destined to accomplish in this lifetime. Longevity is an important factor in living a fulfilled life; the average lifespan for human beings should be anywhere between 120 and 150 years. While I was in Dominica, a woman had just died at the age of 129. What I learned about her lifestyle and the lifestyle of other centenarians is that they led active lives connected to Nature. Dominica is known as the "Nature Island of the Caribbean." Due to its mountainous terrain, very little modern development has occurred and, as a result, most of the population is connected to Nature for their daily needs. This is, of course, a blessing and the way Nature intended for us to live: garden our vegetables and pick fruit off the trees and vines, bathe in her rivers and streams, walk from here to there and everywhere and, most importantly, get an ample amount of sunlight. This simple way of life will add another lifetime to the present lifespan of the average person. That is my ideal of paradise living and health.

Living in the city requires one to take up daily meditation, yoga and/or qi gong, along with one's dietary regimen. The first thing we lose living in an urban environment is oxygen. Therefore, we must do more in the way of breathing exercises to offset this dilemma. What becomes necessary is to retreat every so often to areas away from the city, where there is an abundance of greenery. I believe that this is the most critical aspect to good health and longevity—communing with nature.

Technology, with its many arms, has a hand in almost everything we do and how we live. From communication to entertainment to even the food that we eat, modern technological "advances" have something to do with it. Even the computer upon which I type is a result of this ever-increasing dependency on technology. The convenience of technology comes at the expense of excess radiation and overstimulation. As a result, the human race has become dumbed down and more toxic from an array of daily contact with microwaves, cell phones, smart phones, flat screen televisions, GPS devices, i-everything (pods, pads, phones, books), computers, video games, and hot spots (just to name a few). One thing is certain: the technology trend will increase; there will be more "advances," more "inventions," and more toxic devices in the future.

The devices we use are one thing, but what about the genetically modified food, better named genetic freak food. Genetic freak food, along with modern toxic devices that we come across daily, is a recipe for a genetically freakish race of people. Along with vaccines, drugs, and surgery, there would seem to be no hope for our future. Is more technology worth the expense to our collective health and the environment? Certainly our present health and the survival of future generations are key, but what is more important, is our connection with Nature. The movie *Avatar* (2009) painted a fantastical view of that connection; a worship of what is real and what is Nature and all of its facets. Our connection to Nature should have a religious fervency.

There is a place for religion and religious practice in society. Many churches, temples, and synagogues serve as places of worship for families and individuals to strengthen each other with respect to particular core beliefs and/ or teachings. Religious communities can serve to offset negative behaviors, such as crime, drug abuse, violence, and other ills of society. What about the ills of technology? What about the ills of genetically modified organisms (GMO) as a result of biotechnology? A religious connection to Nature is not necessary, but would certainly provide a platform for connecting what all indigenous cultures around the world did at some point. Their connection meant their survival. Our connection to this modern tech-driven world is presently a slow painful demise for most people and their health and could be a mass wipeout of our human race, if this trend continues.

What is encouraging is the number of movements that reconnect us with Nature. The Green movement is alive and thriving within our concrete jungles. Green products, green construction, green politics, and green festivals have made a difference. Is it enough? The raw food movement has made a difference for thousands of people around the world. Eating all or mostly raw organic food ties us directly to Nature. By eating *Her* food in its natural living state for an extended time, we become a living reflection of what Nature is. Disease has no choice but to disappear. The raw food movement and other positive Nature driven movements are signs that people are waking up to what our potential could be.

Vitamin D, the Sunshine vitamin, has become a hot supplement with naturopaths and nutritionists. Super health blogger, Dr. Mercola, devotes a lot of his blog space to the promotion of Vitamin D for good reason. Science supports the reported health benefits. From a philosophical-spiritual standpoint, the Sun (being the biggest star in our solar system) is the reason life exists. Connecting with the Sun on a daily basis is essential for obvious reasons. It reconnects us to probably the most important component of Nature.

Along with Vitamin D, Vitamin "G" (for Grounding) is on the horizon as the next new health fad. Grounding or Earthing is connecting physically with the Earth. The Earth is a negatively-charged yin (feminine principle) that allows balance within the body for the positively charged yang (male principle) atmosphere by having an antioxidant effect. By wearing rubber or plastic soled shoes, we don't connect with the Earth, and it has a detrimental effect on our health. Ongoing studies and research have shown that grounding reduces inflammation and pain, improves sleep, increases energy, normalizes the body's biological rhythms, improves blood pressure, relieves muscle tensions and headaches, lessons hormonal and menstrual symptoms, and dramatically speeds healing.

There are a number of Earthing products presently on the market and more are sure to come with increased awareness. However, one does not need commercial products to walk barefoot through a garden, or to swim in Nature's rivers, lakes, or oceans. You can benefit from Earthing by getting your hands and feet "dirty." The Sun (male/father) and Earth (female/mother) together and the daily connection for humans and our health mean balance, creation, and completion—life itself.

Increasingly, natural health "discoveries" are in the news, and it can be simply said that all of it relates to reconnecting back to our Mother, Mother Nature. The reverence of religious practices devoted to what is all around us is reason for living (Sun, Earth, Food, Shelter). At one point, it was according to Nature and harmony with Nature's laws. I personally believe on a mass psyche level that it will take a Christian's devotion to Jesus or a Muslim's devotion to Allah for the planet to heal and detox from all the blocks of modern-day living. However, just like people, it usually takes trauma to change. The Earth will be here long after we are gone, but will our future generations enjoy and thrive with the priceless benefits that Nature itself has to give or will they toil in a techno-materialistic polluted world?

Ultimately, the purpose of this book is to establish a consistent fasting regimen that is a part of your life for the rest of your life. Fasting is an art and a good habit that keeps food in perspective. Overindulging in food becomes a sin. Your body can sustain its energy simply when undo energy is not exerted via a constant cycle of food digestion. Rest is equivalent to rejuvenation. If we are eating three meals a day, every day, year after year for our entire lives, then the body has to cure the eventual healing crisis. Disease or illness is created as a way to force you to fast and rest the digestive system. Regular fasting at key points during the year (solstices and equinoxes) and eliminating the breakfast meal from the equation gives the body sufficient rest. The effectiveness of the digestive organs will likely minimize a health crisis. By getting all of our nourishment from a liquid source, the body is able to draw more oxygen from the juices. In addition, when the body does not have to deal with fiber, there is more room and freedom to breathe and, therefore, more oxygen. A yoga practice with deep breathing exercises combined with fasting becomes an ideal combination where beneficial change can happen throughout the body.

Lastly, in analyzing the history of people who lived long lives free from diseases, I believe that the common factors among them lie in their ability to sustain their vitality through moderate eating. It is always a good idea to be conscious of the size of your meal portions. Set a goal after a long fast to reduce your meal portions about 20-50% of what they are presently. Overeating, even with fruits and vegetables, will produce mucus. Between periods of fasting, a proper feasting regimen with the correct combinations of food, in moderation, will have you on the fast track to a long and healthy life.

MUCUS AND DISEASE

What is mucus? Mucus is decomposed blood. Decomposed blood is pus. The actual presence, of mucus within the body is in direct correlation to the manifestation of disease in the body. Whether there is a current feeling of sickness, mucus will eventually present itself in one form or another, continually accumulating from daily habits of eating mucus-forming addictive food. What we see as disease, such as premature aging, cancer, tumors, fibroids, dandruff, and overall breakdown of the human body is really from the layering and accumulation of mucus from most of our lives.

Mucus is a blessing, as much as it is a curse. Without the body's ability to produce mucus, our bodies would not be able to withstand the decades of abuse we put it through from improper feasting. It begins on the day we are born, in most cases with man-made infant "formulas" and vaccinations. When a baby is prematurely weaned off the mother's breast, what usually follows is the first introduction to food via cooked starches. Instead of the sweet nectar of mangos, berries, or bananas as a delightful, clean, and nourishing first food for the infant's gentle digestive lining, the baby instead gets a rice or cereal concoction. This immediately results in the body putting up its mucus defensive protective forces to properly deal with processed foods. Due to the dietary choices for the child by its caregivers, it is not coincidental that a child who has been given these foods and has been prematurely weaned off the mother's milk is plagued by a constant runny nose, nagging cough, wheezing breath, allergies, eczema, and other health issues. Most of us grow into adolescence and adulthood never knowing what it would be like to not have the over-accumulation of mucus plaguing our daily lives.

The effective removal of excess mucus is an extremely daunting task and requires years, if not decades, of disciplined scientific fasting and feasting throughout the rest of one's life. I like to use the analogy of removing crust and slime from cookware made up of encrusted grease and slime from animal flesh, mock meats, starch, and other high mucus-forming foods. A typical approach to cleaning cookware such as this is to first soak the dish in warm water. Soaking dishes in preparation to washing them later is like placing the body on a water or juice fast. The dishes in this analogy represent our physical body and its organs. When we bring in Mother Nature's juices from coconut and citrus fruits, it is analogous to bringing in water well-equipped with its own detergent. When there is an attempt to fast on plain water, it is like trying to wash dishes with no detergent.

After the soaking phase is completed, we have now "loosened" the crust on our pan, or the mucus residues in our bodies, and we are now ready to scrub it clean. The scrubbing action that takes place in our bodies is done by the food we ingest after the fast. The food used to break a fast is as equally important as the juice used during the fast. Breaking the fast on incorrect food can be disastrous. The first meal should consist of a high moisture fruit, such as watermelon. The fiber in the melon will provide the scrub to remove loosened mucus in the digestive track. When breaking a fast, dried fruit such as dates, raisins and mangos, should be avoided. Optimal foods to break a fast are explained in further detail in the Fasting Regimen of the program.

As we approach a fasting and detox regimen, putting everything into proper perspective, the idea of ridding our bodies of a lifetime of waste accumulation for most of us can appear daunting, especially if we have arrived at a point where our body has regressed to a debilitating condition. Diseases such as cancer, heart attack, stroke, diabetes, hypertension, thyroid issues, chronic fatigue, arthritis, asthma, short life span, balding, and grey hair are just the body's reaction in dealing with mucus over many decades of violation of the body temple.

Nevertheless, the way that life works is that our worst moments present the opportunity to experience our best and most unforgettable moments. In order for us to reach new levels of personal growth, we take quantum leaps when we choose to make the best out of what may appear to be the worst situation of our lives.

Understanding that most, if not all of us, have a lifetime of waste accumulation in our bodies, a proper feasting and fasting regimen is a habitual journey that has no end destination. The ultimate goal is to feel a glimpse of the possibility of what our human potential could be. I often visualize what it was like for our ancient ancestors who all ate a paradise diet without cooking and "modern" agriculture. I am sure that there was a harmony that existed within their bodies (physical, emotional, and spiritual) which, therefore, extended into their relationships, families, extended families and communities. To live in such harmony is my dream for all human beings. Whether a paradise communal living situation will happen in my present lifetime or in some future generation, I feel that the human spirit will at some point overtake our present disconnection from paradise living.

"You are what you eat" is the old timeless saying; I prefer to say, "You eat what you are." What we eat is dictated by what we are craving. If you are overloaded with mucus, your cravings will generate a desire to keep eating high mucus-forming foods. Your brain, in which mucus also is present, will influence and even dominate your thoughts to keep the high mucus-forming foods coming. It's a serious addiction that results in a downward spiral of our health and vitality.

To break the cycle, a complete examination of one's diet, lifestyle practices, occupations, and family life has to be looked at to see which adjustments need to be made. When I'm doing consultations with clients, I begin from birth, because the body has a memory of everything it ever consumed. Life's circumstances also will dictate when a change is necessary. A traumatic event can be the best opportunity to begin a new life course. Food can cloud and complicate judgment.   Fasting brings clarity and peace. With the information contained in this book, a blueprint with insight is provided, showing the steps to take for success.   It is of vital importance to journal your progress and your body's every feeling and to continually note any changes with each fast.   The goal is to feel increasingly better and take larger strides on your never-ending glorious journey of paradise living.

ANOTHER LOOK AT GERM THEORY

Modern day society is very conscious about germs. We are all taught from the very beginning to always wash our hands and practice many other daily outer hygienic practices, along with keeping our living environments sanitary and clean. This is great as well as vital. In working with food every day, there is also a proper code of hygiene and sanitation that goes with the production of food. Taking into account this high consciousness of cleanliness that is present within our society, one would think that no one would fall victim to the result of a germ entering the body and wreaking havoc; however, this is not the case. The pharmaceutical industry is doing well in the production of antibiotics, drugs, vaccines and other over-the-counter poisons that are either supposed to eliminate the germ that is causing problems in your body or bring it under control. Now, let me begin by saying I am no biologist, nor do I think I need to be one in order to analyze this subject. I am just an observer of life; one who strives to live as close to Mother Nature's laws as possible, in an environment that doesn't respect Mother Nature.

Germ Theory proposes that microorganisms naked to the human eye that originate outside of the human organism are the cause of many diseases. It is my assertion that most, if not all, diseases are the result of improper dietary hygiene and not germs from someone else or some other mysterious entity. There is a saying that sums it up perfectly, "You don't catch a cold, you eat one." First and foremost, by taking this approach, if you fall victim to disease, you and you alone are taking full responsibility for your present diseased condition and not passing that responsibility to a mysterious germ entity that was passed to you by your neighbor, your cousin, or even your mate. I personally like the idea of taking full responsibility for anything that may harm me, whether it is disease, misfortune, or other adverse circumstances. Certainly with conditions relative to our health and body temples, we have to look first at the fuel used and determine whether it was in balance. Any aspect of ingestion could throw the body into a healing crisis. You could eat the wrong foods at the wrong time. You could eat too much. You could eat foods that are out of season. These and many more situations that involve imbalanced food intake could put the body off kilter. Mass media indoctrination and popular misbeliefs will have most people jumping to the conclusion that a germ invader got them, only to correctly find out that their imbalanced food intake was responsible.

Let us examine the food we eat and how food creates disease. All foods, with the exception of fruits and green leafy vegetables, create mucus in the body. The mucus lining is the first line of internal defense that the body has against improper food and toxic substances that are put into the body. Without the mucus lining, we would not live very long. Even raw soaked nuts and seeds will create mucus. For most human beings who are not breastfed and/or who receive vaccinations begin the process of mucus accumulation at birth. We have all seen formula-fed babies with runny noses all too often. If you were formula fed or began with the rice cereal (or other high mucus-forming foods) as some of your first food, the reality is that mucus is still present in your body system!

I think it is safe to say that most of us have eaten mucus-laden foods for most of our lives, whether we followed a vegetarian or vegan diet from birth or a Muslim (Halal) diet with no pork or red meat. An over-accumulation of mucus in the body forces the body to eliminate mucus in an infinite number of ways. Common mucus elimination methods used by the body are: excretion through the body organs; internally through the lungs (common cold); colon (diarrhea, foul-smelling stool); stomach (nausea, vomiting, ulcers); brain (headache); externally through the skin (pimples, eczema, dandruff, fungus, foul odors, rash); and eyes (morning mucus). Ultimately, if there is no significant change or check in the diet and lifestyle, the degree of disease, pain and suffering will escalate to a higher level after decades of bodily abuse, causing cancer, diabetes, stroke, hypertension, thyroid issues, heart trouble, tumors, and arthritis. Now that we clearly see the connection between mucus and diseases, how can we intelligently consider germ theory as a viable theory at all?

Given our paranoia with germs, we should be more conscious about the foods that are put into our bodies. One of the first things we do to eliminate germs is wash our hands, which takes fresh running water. Compare this to the process of eating. The first question that should be asked before putting any food into our mouths is how much water is contained in this food? Most fruits will contain 70-90% water; equally, the body is made up of at least 70% water. Take a daily journal of your food intake and see how much of the food you eat contains at least 70% water. Most health conscious people will either have fruit for breakfast or as a snack between meals. We need to begin to make fruit THE MEAL itself and not just a small part of the meal. It's not healthy to eat two or three meals in which the natural living water and enzymes have been cooked out, reduced to less than 20 or 10% water, and then drink a gallon of water or juice behind it. This is not proper and not natural. Natural food that contains mostly water is CLEAN food. Clean food allows clean blood cells to permeate and nourish all the body's systems and allows the colon to work perfectly every time without the elimination of foul smelling stools. When you pass stool, it should not take 30-45 minutes before the next person can enter the bathroom!

Eating primarily clean food will have an impact on other outer hygienic practices, such as the use of deodorant, soap, and sanitizer. The use of these products should decrease to a large degree if the primary make up of your food is high water content fruits and vegetables. Because of air pollution and other environmental toxins from urban living, it is very important to bathe daily. However, under different circumstances, such as a clean (nontoxic) environment coupled with a clean diet, it may not be necessary.

When I think about wild animal life, I ask myself, "Do they wash their hands?" "Do they wash their food before eating?" Maybe they do, maybe they don't, but definitely not to the degree that humans do. You would think that, given our belief in germs, that germs and bacteria would have exterminated wild animals long ago. Given our sanitary practices versus animals in the wild, we are out of sync and wild animals are in sync with the way Mother Nature intended. Wild animals experience nothing but divine health.

How do we attack a lifetime of mucus accumulation in the body's entire being? There is only one true way, and it is not with colonics, herbs, homeopathy, essential oils, or other supplements. These methods mentioned are very effective; however, they are all secondary measures to scientific fasting, diet, and lifestyle. A colonic can be effective in removing mucoid plaque in your colon, but it will not reach the mucus stored in the brain or the eyes or all other parts of your body. The same holds true for homeopathic remedies and herbs; they work with your body to attack disease symptoms, yet the latent mucus remains throughout your body. Through periodic scientific fasting, your body works to slowly eliminate mucus from all parts of the body and internal organs. After the first day of fasting, by examining the mucus layer on your tongue, the thickness of mucus on the tongue becomes the barometer of how much mucus is stored internally throughout the body.

Germs do exist in our toxic society; however, the presence of germs does not replace the fact that our diet and lifestyle are the primary reason we are not divinely healthy. Germ theory is barely even 150 years old, yet human life existed long before that. Nonetheless, germ theory has become the foundation for not only allopathic doctors but naturopaths and alternative healers, as well. The germ theory is at best just a theory. Our ancient ancestors knew that proper diet, periodic fasting, sunlight, yoga, and qi gong practices equated to divine health and longevity. The propaganda machine will continue to feed us the paranoia of germs to support their money-making industries, from drugs to vaccines to hand sanitizers. We must challenge our false cravings, the propaganda and emotionally-driven diets. Start fasting, and make it a permanent part of your lifestyle.

The ultimate goal is to fast and wake up the next day with a clear tongue. Until that happens, disease is present in your body in a latent (inactive) state. Waking up with a clear tongue after fasting is the only indicator that a lifetime of mucus accumulation is removed from your body. This can take years, maybe more than a decade, depending on the level of toxicity in the body. With practice and consistency, you can become a master faster and your own doctor, as the body was designed to self-heal with the proper application of periodic fasting.

SOLAR HEAT IS A HEALER

With the cycle of spring and summer, the heat turns up as the Earth tilts, so that the Northern Hemisphere is in closer proximity to the Sun's nurturing solar rays. If you are not living in an equatorial region of the world, then that means the late spring, summer, and early fall in the Northern Hemisphere present an opportunity for healing.

We rarely allow the Sun, the largest star in our solar system, to come in contact and bless our skin on a daily basis and allow it to provide valuable nutrients and stimulating melanin production. Sun and Air are the invisible foods. Too much time is spent indoors. Ideally, we should be spending close to 100% of our time outdoors! Many activities, which are exclusively done indoors, could or should be done outdoors like sleeping, bathing, and even childbirth. The crazy thing about our society is that we will confine ourselves indoors when we are ill, often times in the worst places, like hospitals. People who live in non-tropical regions are faced with challenges that can compromise their health and longevity.

The intense summer heat in the urban cities around the world means an overuse of air conditioning. You can literally never experience fresh air during the summer when air conditioning is everywhere—in homes, cars, and workplaces.

Modern cave-like convenience has become the modern day tragedy for our health. We have become today's cavemen, going from our "comfortable" air-conditioned house to our air-conditioned car, to our air-conditioned office. Do you realize that in order for our modern caves to be kept cool, air conditioners have to blow hot air into the environment? This, of course, can lead to temperatures becoming unusually high. If the heat is uncomfortable for you, then it is likely a sign that you have a high level of toxins in your system. Eighty and even ninety degree Fahrenheit temperatures should be comfortable. The opportunity to sweat is also welcoming. It wouldn't be a bad idea to have a good sweat every day. Saunas, hot yoga, and heated spa treatments are very healing because heat facilitates movement. The heat begins to loosen toxins that are stagnant in the body. Toxins, beginning to move, can be very uncomfortable; you unconsciously turn on the air-conditioning, and; therefore, allow toxins to remain stagnant in your body. There goes a detoxification opportunity lost!

Heated indoor environments are good, but they do not replace heat generated by the Sun. Solar heat is most concentrated at the equator. It is no coincidence that the greatest and most valuable resources exist in and around the equatorial regions of the world where the sun's rays are strongest, from food, oil, and metals to precious stones and minerals. The best tasting tropical foods are found there. When you are eating tropical fruits, you are really eating the tropical Sun. Just being in a tropical environment facilitates energy, better health, and longevity. Just ask old retirees who have relocated to warmer climates.

The closer you move towards the equator, the greater the amount of food choices and, hence, the greater amount of food resources. When we consider detoxification, the food growing closest to the sun on the highest palm is, of course, coconuts. Therefore, coconuts are carrying the greatest level of the sun's healing energy and will facilitate the greatest amount of movement in the body's internal organs when taken alone as a fast.

By allowing the sun on our person, on our physical naked body, we are receiving the ultimate food. Along with Vitamin D, the sun provides photosynthetic nourishment for the body. Clothes, sunglasses, umbrellas and sunscreen all impede the direct, invaluable sun energy-body connection. By having an up-close and personal relationship with the sun, we should, ideally, lose our appetite for physical food.

Do the best you can to take advantage of the summertime Sun. It is beneficial to not only have the sun bless your skin but your eyes and, especially, your hair. Sunlight on your hair will stimulate chlorophyll production in your body the same way that chlorophyll is produced in green leaves on trees. That is why green leafy vegetables are not as critical if you are getting plenty of sun. Now, go outside and get some SUN!

STARCH + SOY = VEGETARIAN DIET

From my late teenage years to my early twenties, I made the transition from omnivore to vegetarian, eliminating red meat, chicken, fish, and dairy products. Soy was believed to be healthier, and it was exciting to experience all the soy substitutes for meat and dairy.

Growing up, I learned from followers of Islam that pork was to be shunned because the pig was the filthiest animal. If you ate swine, then you would be infected with very dangerous parasites. Muslim propaganda inspired many health conscious people to move from completely omnivorous eating to eliminating not only pork, but all red meat and dairy. Eating fish and fowl was thought to be healthier and, if you went a step further to eliminate all animal products, a very likely substitution would be soy and soy by-products. The interesting irony is that while pork was demonized, soy was praised as a great cholesterol-free protein rich substitute for meat and dairy. It was only after making the transition to raw foods that I realized how powerful and addictive the "healthy" cooked, starchy vegetarian foods were. Eliminating "healthy" chips, cereal, wheat, popcorn, oats, beans, cookies, donuts, bread, biscuits, cornbread, pasta, rice, and cakes was my last and most difficult hurdle to following a truly healthy diet.

Using soy as a foundation food is where modern day vegetarianism or veganism fails. Soy is simply not a food to use as a staple for fat and protein needs. In fact, just the opposite is true. Eating a significant amount of soy products can lead to a number of health issues. A number of studies have shown cases of hormonal disruptions, thyroid problems, evidence of inhibitors that block mineral assimilation and absorption, cancer, infertility, and miscarriage for women, and loss of libido and erectile dysfunction for men.

Eliminating pork and red meat products was relatively simple in terms of identifying what is pork. There are always exceptions which may contain by-products and not be so obvious, for example, Jello. Soy and its by-products are very pervasive throughout all processed foods. Buy a salad dressing or a sauce marinade, and it will likely have soy and/or rapeseed oil. What's worse, given that 95% of all soy is genetically engineered, odds are that when you are eating veggie burgers, soy mock meats or french fries, not only are you ingesting dangerous levels of soy oil and protein, but you are also ingesting genetically-engineered viruses.

For a true vegetarian, what are the optimal sources for protein and fat? Eating fruits and salads is nice but, ideally, it always comes down to balance. Great sources of vegetarian fat and protein are from nuts, coconuts, seeds, avocados, olives and ackee (popular in Jamaica). These are some examples of foods that should be staples for our healthy fat and protein sources. We need fats and protein, as well as sugar. Healthy food is food in its natural balanced state.

Sixty years ago, soy and other vegetable oils replaced more costly coconut and palm oils. Coconut and palm oils came from tropical regions, and soy oil could be produced more locally in seasonal environments. Deceptive marketing demonized coconut and palm oils for being high in saturated fat. Conversely, soy, corn, and rapeseed oils were being touted as "healthy." Cattle ranchers in the 1940s discovered that when their cattle were fed tropical palm oils, the cattle didn't gain weight; in fact, they were lean, active and hungry. When the ranchers fed their cattle soy and corn products, it had an anti-thyroid effect and, as a result, the cattle gained more weight on less food. Soy protein curds, such as tofu and bean curd, were by-products of soy oil and were also marketed as a health food. It is critical to understand that Asians traditionally ate soy using sophisticated fermenting techniques that allowed the soy to have nutritional value, by reducing or eliminating all inhibitors present. It is the inhibitors in soy that makes it a lethal dangerous food.

As the veil on the dangers of soy continues to be lifted, continue to do your research and determine for yourself and your family what is the best dietary regimen. Remember, more nutritional forms of soy are always fermented, and they include tempeh, natto, miso, and soy sauce. Tofu, bean curd, veggie burgers, and TVP should be avoided or limited for optimal vibrancy.

Cooked starches are the most addictive food on the planet. You could argue that cooked starches fall in the same category as all addictive drugs.

72

In fact, it is no different from over-the-counter drugs or recreational drugs when looking at the long-term damaging effects on the body. As a whole, cooked processed starches raise the blood glucose sugar more than any other food. This drug-like effect is addictive and dangerous. Besides, cooked starch is the main reason for improper food combinations. Anytime anyone eats cooked starch for a snack or a meal, it is almost always combined with another food, such as fat, that the body cannot digest simultaneously. If you eat starches by themselves, they are more exposed for the food that they actually are: a paste. It is dangerous to combine starches with oil, butter, cream, cheese, gravy, milk, or icing. It leads to improper digestion and poor assimilation, which will then lead to weight gain and more serious complications.

It should be mentioned that the processed starches we find in many foods today are again a result of the devolution of agribusiness and its adverse impact on our health. Wheat flour devolved as a result of removing key components of the plant which were cooked and processed for the purpose of increasing its shelf life. The greater a food's shelf life, the shorter your life! Starches also are devoid of any color. The color of food is very important and critical for nutrients and minerals. Usually, the richer the pigment, the richer the nutritional content. Starches have no nutritional content in comparison to dark berries and green leafy vegetables.

Starches are absent of any moisture. Because they lack moisture, beans, rice, barley and oats require boiling just to chew them. After starches are boiled to add moisture content, fat usually is added to these foods to make them more palatable. Healthy fatty plant foods such as avocado, olives, nuts, and seeds do not lead to weight gain. It is the combination of starch with fat that leads to weight gain and more serious complications down the road.

Starch is an acid-forming food. The acid present in starchy grain foods is carbonic acid. Over time, the liver will turn as hard as a piece of wood. Stones will develop in the gall bladder and kidneys. Other common complications include hypertension, diabetes, hemorrhoids, tumors and cancer.

The only solution to beating the crack-like addiction to cooked starch is by eating raw green leafy vegetables. Kale, collards, spinach, dandelion, watercress, and arugula should replace beans, rice, pasta, bread, and barley. Greens are alkaline and are highly mineralized. If you replace rice with kale, you will create another layer of health, vitality, true nourishment, and fulfillment. Green juices and smoothies are great, but I believe it is of tantamount importance to chew your greens raw and, as often as possible, without dressings and sweeteners. This will exercise and re-mineralize your teeth and help to change the chemistry of your blood and body from a toxic acid to a healing alkaline environment.

After 20 years of practicing the vegetarian lifestyle, with the last 10 being raw, I have come to the realization that if you are not doing at least an 80% raw food diet, then your diet is not healthy. The raw vegetarian foods include fruits, vegetables, nuts, seeds, sprouts, flowers, and herbs. For vegetarians/vegans who are not making the aforementioned foods their primary foods, then the primary filler foods for them are likely soy and cooked starches, which will undoubtedly lead to disease and premature death.

Since business dictates what is largely available, becoming vegetarian has become relatively simple with the abundance of mock cheese and meat items. However, if we want to do better, being vegetarian is not where we should be comfortable. The mock substitutions for a carnivorous diet are usually a soy or gluten derivative. Foremost, soy is not a health food; gluten for that matter is just as bad. Soy, having its origins from Asia, was not originally consumed in high quantities as it is consumed today. The following excerpts are from www.soyonlineservice.co.nz:

In short, not that much, and contrary to what the industry may claim, soy has never been a staple in Asia. A study of the history of soy use in Asia shows that it was used by the poor during times of extreme food shortage, and only then the soybeans were carefully prepared (e.g., by lengthy fermentation) to destroy the soy toxins. Yes, the Asians understood soy alright!

Many vegetarians in the USA and Europe and Australasia would think nothing of consuming 8 ounces (about 220 grams) of tofu and a couple of glasses of soy milk per day, two or three times a

76

week. But, this is well in excess of what Asians typically consume; they generally use small portions of soy to complement their meal. It should also be noted that soy is not the main source of dietary protein and that a regime of calcium-set tofu and soy milk bears little resemblance to the soy consumed traditionally in Asia.

The following is taken from The Weston A. Price Foundation's website www.westonaprice.org, a nonprofit organization that is dedicated to restoring nutrient dense food to the human diet through education, research and activism, on the dangers of soy:

High levels of phytic acid in soy reduce assimilation of calcium, magnesium, copper, iron and zinc. Phytic acid in soy is not neutralized by ordinary preparation methods, such as soaking, sprouting and long, slow cooking. High phytate diets have caused growth problems in children.

Trypsin inhibitors in soy interfere with protein digestion and may cause pancreatic disorders. In test animals soy containing trypsin inhibitors caused stunted growth.

Soy phytoestrogens disrupt endocrine function and have the potential to cause infertility and to promote breast cancer in adult women.

Soy phytoestrogens are potent antithyroid agents that cause hypothyroidism and may cause thyroid cancer. In infants, consumption of soy formula has been linked to autoimmune thyroid disease.

Vitamin B12 analogs in soy are not absorbed and increase the body's requirement for B12.

Soy foods increase the body's requirement for vitamin D.

Fragile proteins are denatured during high temperature processing to make soy protein isolate and textured vegetable protein.

Processing of soy protein results in the formation of toxic lysinoalanine and highly carcinogenic nitrosamines.

Free glutamic acid or MSG, a potent neurotoxin, is formed during soy food processing and additional amounts are added to many soy foods.

Soy foods contain high levels of aluminum which is toxic to the nervous system and the kidneys.

Soy is extremely toxic. Many vegans following a vegetarian diet will have major health crises by consuming soy on a daily basis. Case in point, Aveline Kushi, founder of the macrobiotic diet (a vegetarian diet high in starch and soy and low in fat), died of cancer. Her daughter died of cancer as well. If you are vegetarian and you eat a lot of mock meats and starches, you, as with most vegetarians of today, are following what is similar to what was defined as the macrobiotic diet.

How did this happen to promoters and leaders of a vegetarian movement? It's very simple. Starch and soy are toxic to our bodies, period. Both are high mucus formers. When we uncover the root of all diseases, we usually find mucus (not germs) as the primary culprit. Germs are the end result of mucus. How does cancer connect with mucus? Cancer is an advanced organized stage of decades of mucus being continually formed in the body. Years or decades of mucus being formed in the body will ultimately lead to cancer, whether or not you are vegetarian. Therefore, being vegetarian or eating largely soy and starchy foods is not healthy. These foods should be eaten minimally or not at all for excellent health.

Our food choices should largely consist of fresh foods in the form of fruits and greens. Fruits and greens should be the primary staples, with nuts, seeds and sprouted grains eaten occasionally. This food regimen makes up the fruitarian diet, and we are all fruitarians whether we choose to eat that way or not. Congratulations if you don't eat any animal flesh. However, if at least two out of every three meals consist of soy and starch, I ask you to do better and make at least one meal a day all fruit, and your second meal all greens with either fruits or nuts. If two-thirds of your meals within a day are fresh, you are on the right track to attaining the highest level of health.

SUPPLEMENTS: ARE THEY NECESSARY?

Walk into any health food store today and you will find your typical aisles of food organized with fresh produce, bulk bins, canned and jarred goods, and frozen foods. What has emerged in more recent times, especially in today's health food store, is the supplement section. Health supplements have replaced your typical over-the-counter medicines, such as Tylenol and Robitussin. The supplement section has literally become a store within a store. Every supplement section within a health food store has specially trained staff, armed with information to sell you the next magic health pill. The government, corporate America, and the powers that be (i.e., the FDA) have taken notice as supplements have become big business, a $27 BILLION dollar business in 2010 alone. As health seekers, we need to ask certain questions: Are supplements necessary? Will supplements make a difference in my health? If I do decide to take supplements, what would be the best supplements to take?

Supplement sales are certain to continue, barring government intervention, as health entrepreneurs and clientele alike appreciate the convenience of popping a pill or a capsule, mixing a protein powder or a liquid supplement into a smoothie. No matter how "good" one's supplement is, the "difference maker" will always be changing one's diet and eliminating addictive harmful foods. There can be a place for supplementation in one's dietary regimen, but it is low on the totem pole. If I had to rank the tenants of a great health practice, diet would be number one, fasting two, exercise three, emotional poise four, and a good supplemental regimen will be somewhere between 6 and 10.

A dietary supplement, as defined by Congress in the Dietary Supplement Health and Education Act in 1994, is a product that 1) is intended to supplement the diet, and 2) contains one or more dietary ingredients (including vitamins; minerals; herbs or other botanicals, amino acids, and other substances) or their constituents. What is a dietary supplement really? A supplement can be considered a partial part of FOOD that is usually used to compliment one's dietary needs or to provide temporary relief during a health crisis by over-stimulating the body.

Similar to other secondary healing practices, such as a colonic, taking and depending upon supplements can be a psychological crutch. A psychological health crutch is a healing practice that improperly replaces what will make the difference in the mind of the individual. For example, a colonic can give someone the false idea that they are being cleaned out; therefore, they don't have to change their diet. Supplements, which can be herbal powders, herbal teas, herbal tinctures, homeopathic remedies, essential oils, therapeutic enzymes, or green "superfood" powders, are all products which can be effective, but only if one's diet is sound. Supplements can be the crutch that allows one to not change his/her diet and, instead, to depend on the temporary stimulation that any supplement will provide if there is a health crisis.

The body is always remaking itself out of the raw materials that one is continually eating. Therefore, diet and fasting will always be the primary factors in good health and longevity. We can look at the contribution that a supplement makes by breaking down our daily intake of a particular supplement in mathematical proportion to one's daily caloric intake of food. If I am eating 2000 calories per day in food and my daily vitamin supplement is contributing 10 out of 2000 calories, which amounts to less than a 1% contribution to my health. These supplements can be quite expensive for only a 1% contribution! If we consider whether our supplements are contributing less than 1% to our health but 10 - 20% of our food budget, then we need to reevaluate how we spend our money.

Understand that there can be a place for supplementation if and only if our diet is sound and our budget allows. It will never replace diet, exercise, and periodic fasting unless you are having meals of supplements, like a supplement salad.

FASTING IS A LIFESTYLE PRACTICE

What are you good at? Is it your job, a particular hobby or art form? We all become good at behaviors that are done repeatedly; it is our habitual behavior that transforms us into the individuals that we are and that we hope to become. As far as our health, longevity, and well-being, what are we doing habitually that is continually cultivating a sound mind, body, and soul?

Our health is the foundation for all wealth. Our physical body is the house for our spiritual being and, without a sound body, nothing else matters—not your assets, your bank account, your physical possessions, or even your family and community when your health is compromised. When we determine and fully understand that the nature of disease is the lifelong accumulation of toxic waste matter from addictive "food," we can take action to really come into the paradise of vitality. We must systematically fast as a continual practice.

In this age of information, the consciousness of the human race is growing at light speed. In that growing awareness is the understanding of eating better, organic food, and eco-living. We have seen businesses with increased consciousness, such as Whole Foods, become a major supermarket chain in this country. We have also seen thousands and maybe millions of people adopt a vegetarian lifestyle, and even a completely raw food diet. This being said, it is my firm belief that scientific fasting has to be a part of anyone's program for the attainment of higher health.

Health food supplements, herbal and homeopathic remedies, natural remedies such as colonics, massage, acupuncture, acupressure, and other healing modalities, are fantastic ways of dealing with health crises. Awareness of these remedies is replacing allopathic drugs and irreversible surgical procedures. However, fasting, when done scientifically and continually as a lifestyle practice, is the best.

Two principle ideas make fasting superior. The first is that the body is designed to self-heal. By doing colonics, Smooth Move herbal teas and other "cleansing" supplements, you are saying that your body is not capable of doing the work itself. Sometimes we do need help in the form of a tea or colonic. However, ultimately, teas and colonics handicap our own internal organs and become a crutch just as with any other crutch. We have to earn our good health and well-being. Fasting and proper feasting allow our stomach, intestines, liver and kidneys to become increasingly stronger, along with a good yoga practice.

The second principle is that the nature and root of all disease stems from a lifetime of layered mucus or pus that is in every cell, every organ (not just the colon) and every fiber in our body. The ONLY way to deal with this fact is to fast and fast continually. Each time we fast, our body removes a thin layer of waste that is present everywhere in our body. With each fast, it becomes easier. Your internal organs become stronger, and your detox reactions are lessened. We should all aspire to eliminate all mucus from our bodies!

I personally feel that the fasting process should be fun, something that can be enjoyed while giving up the foods that we crave. This is part of the reason why a major aspect of the fast that we supervise involves drinking Mother Nature's water, the coconut water, which is naturally sweet and healing. It removes waste matter without the use of herbal teas and colonics or enemas. Sugar cane juice is delicious nectar that we can enjoy without guilt on this type of fast. In addition to the sweet, we introduce sour into our juices, such as lime or passion fruit, which becomes a delectable marriage of flavors when combined with sugar cane juice. We can't forget about the greens, because this is where we get our sodium and mineral salts. A typical green juice will have lemon or lime with ginger. This is what paradise fasting is all about.

The question remains, "How long or how many fasts would I have to undergo to completely rid my body of waste, pus and mucus build-up from a lifetime of abuse?" My answer is another lifetime! A lifetime or journey doesn't end with 5 fasts or 500 fasts. Life is never about the destination but the journey. Fasting is a beautiful journey of really getting to know one's true self. All of us have eaten enough food for at least 3 lifetimes. It is time to bring balance to who we are and what we can become. When we embrace and fall in love with the process and journey of healing our temples at the highest level, then we can have the opportunity to cherish the feeling of a higher, blissful life.

Masters of dance, art or business all love and appreciate what they do. When they attain levels of mastery, only then do they begin to know the discipline that has become, for some, a key element of their lives. Let us think of fasting as a lifetime discipline and art form that we can embrace to make us better, healthier, wealthier and happier.

HOW LONG SHOULD YOU FAST?

A common question that comes up is how long should we fast at one particular time? We are all at various levels of toxicity and that always has to be taken into consideration. For most people, a week is safe. To put it in perspective, how would someone who hasn't run for say five or ten years begin to train for a marathon? To do it correctly, so that one prevents injury, you may start with a mile run, and then maybe after a month or two build up to five miles. After three to six months of training, you may now be ready to run five to ten miles at one time. Beyond six months, you are ready for your final phase of training that will prepare you for the ultimate test of running 26 miles. Fasting has to be approached in a similar fashion. I know people who have psyched themselves up to do a 40-day water fast and endured for the 40 days only to end the fast and fail miserably because they did too much too soon. How would most of us do if we went out and ran a marathon right this very second? Even if we completed the 26 miles, we would probably be sore for weeks due to lack of preparation, and we would put our bodies at high risk for injury.

Fasting is no different from any other training and practice. In actuality, fasting should be the foundational training for any and every other discipline that you are undertaking. The fact that it makes you a better you, allows you to gain and reap greater rewards at whatever is already being done. Whether you are relying on your mental abilities, physical abilities, or a combination of the two, with fasting as a consistent practice, you should be more efficient at your job, business, relationships, or physical activity.

My first suggestion would be to master the discipline of fasting one day per week. The particular day of the week should be the same day each week. I would suggest a day that you are normally weak or have low energy. Growing up, I always had low energy on Thursdays. I never understood why, but it remained consistent throughout my life. In contrast, my high energy day was Friday. It may seem like common sense to fast on your high energy day, but this day correlates to a heightened appetite. Given that fasting ideally should allow you to have more energy, it is my recommendation that you fast on your lowest energy day of the week. You also can consider your weekly schedule, because you want any external factors to be supportive and not the opposite. From a planetary perspective, Saturday would be a great day for most people and not just because it is a day of the weekend. Saturday is Saturn's Day, and Saturn astrologically governs structure, discipline and guides us through life's hard lessons. Given the energy of Saturday -- or Saturn's day, -- it is a great day to fast every week. When picking your day of the week to fast, monitor your energy each day and consider your schedule, so that you pick the day that is best for you.

If you are able to fast one day per week every week throughout the year and, hopefully, the rest of your lifetime, everything else you do in your life should be easy. Fasting one day a week is a very difficult skill and habit to maintain. I face each day with the possibility that I may fast or just do high moisture fruits. Doing high moisture fruits would also count in my book as a fast for your fasting day. When discussing fasting as a lifestyle practice, regularly doing just high water fruits, such as melons, citrus, berries or sub-acid fruits, such as pineapple, mango, pears, apples and plums, during an entire day will do wonders for your body temple. The high water content of the fruit will properly nourish your cells, the fiber will stimulate nice movement for your bowels, and the next day you should have a white caked tongue which means that mucus is being moved out of your body.

CYCLICAL FASTING

The universe operates on a continual cycle. Living in this cyclic universe, our bodies are no different. Every minute, hour, day, month, year, and so forth, represents a cycle that will forever repeat itself. Recognizing the cycles of time as they operate through our life and by incorporating the practice of fasting within the appropriate cycle, we are not only healing our bodies, but we are fine-tuning our vibration with the cosmic energy of this universe.

To gain greater insight into cycles, it is a good idea to study the basics of astrology. You should understand your personal astrological cycle, which corresponds to the planetary energies. Consult an astrologer who can draw up your astrological chart and make recommendations for your ideal fasting time. Of course, the solstices and equinoxes present an opportunity for everyone to fast for at least 3 days. During the four seasonal changes of the year, the body goes into an additional detoxification mode by releasing toxins built up in the small intestines. By liquefying our diet with fresh juices or by eating primarily fresh high moisture fruits during this period, we offset the added mucus

95

release of the body, usually seen as allergies, influenza, colds, and other bacterial or viral infections. The added mucus release is offset by allowing the elimination of the body to be more effective. Also, there isn't any additional mucus created by the toxic foods that most people eat.

In addition to knowing when the seasons change, it is paramount to be familiar with the moon cycle. The moon goes through a complete cycle by traveling through the twelve signs of the zodiac every 28 days. It begins with the new moon on the first day of the cycle; by the 14th day, the moon is full and then wanes back to the new moon by the end of the 28-day cycle. As fasting practitioners, we should understand that the moon affects our emotions more than any other planet in our solar system, and our emotions have sister connections with food and the way we eat. Being that our emotions are subject to a monthly or 28-day lunar cycle, we can use this opportunity to fast with the moon's energy.

If you are looking to start a new project or idea, fasting with the new moon, along with an associated meditation will put that project on the "fast" track to manifestation. The frequency of fasting once a month during the lunar cycle is more than ideal. Men and women alike are affected by the gravitational forces of the moon. Fasting with each new moon throughout the year will put your life on a higher energy cosmic vibration.

For women, in particular, the length and intensity of menstruation is in direct correlation to the amount of toxic food that you eat during a particular month. Women can benefit by scheduling a fast around their personal 28-day cycle. It could be planned during menstruation, or it could be during the midpoint of their cycle. Fasting three to seven days per month, every month, will put you on the fast track to paradise health. For those who are overweight and on heavy medications, you may have to work yourself up to a fast. What I recommend in those cases is to do an exclusive raw food diet for 90 days. I should also mention that the Juice Fast is designed so that you have MORE energy, not less. Therefore, you will be able to work more and sleep less. You can be better at your job or business, with your family and mate, and really understand that food in our society does more to get in the way, rather than truly nourish us.

RAISE YOUR BODY'S SENSITIVITY

One of the most common misconceptions about health is the frequency of illness being a measure of one's well-being. For clarity, when I say sick, I mean bedrest and unable to perform your usual daily activities, physical or mental. It is common to hear someone say, "I rarely get sick." Is the frequency of illness a true barometer for our health? Certainly, no one likes the feeling of being ridden with symptoms that force us to stay in bed. If you are one of the fortunate who infrequently gets ill, that may be fine in the short term, but depending on your lifestyle and your habits, you may be setting yourself up for a major illness in the long run.

The body is resilient and adaptable to unfavorable lifestyle changes and habits. Take cigarette smoking as an example. A chain smoker has desensitized him or herself to the point where he or she is now able to withstand a punishing amount of toxic smoke in the body temple on a daily basis. Take another person who has been used to breathing clean unpolluted air and submit him or her to the same assault that the chain smoker is under, and it could likely lead to sudden death. The sensitivity of the non-smoker cannot withstand the suddenness of the impact from poisons to which the chain smoker devolved. Now, is the chain smoker healthier because he or she can withstand more poison? Of course not!

For vegetarians and even raw foodists alike, this principle of sensitivity applies when we are seeking to raise the health of our body temple. Most food will either have a dominant taste of saltiness or sweetness. For most vegetarians who prefer sweet food, the sweet food will usually be a starch. Starchy food is very stimulating and creates a lot of mucus in the body. Starch also is almost always combined with a protein source, which is an improper food combination. When starch and protein are combined with, for example, a veggie burger (bread=starch, soy burger=protein), then that will lead to improper digestion. The starch-protein food combination usually causes gas and, in the long term, leads to more serious digestive issues. Telling on myself for a moment, my vice is definitely salt. Whether it's sea salt, Celtic grey mineral sea salt, Real Salt or even pink salt from deep within the Himalayan Mountains, salt is salt is salt. When using salt, it is definitely preferable to use the aforementioned brands rather than Morton's salt. Salt is a rock that enters the body as salt and leaves the body as salt. Of course, when it comes into the body, it provides much stimulation to the palate and the entire body. This stimulation is very stressful to the body, mainly in the arteries and joints.

About 4 years ago, I was suffering from chronic knee pain. As an aspiring yogi, I was putting significant stress on my knee joints, trying to create the full range of motion in my knee. The pain progressed to the point where for about two months I had to suspend my yoga practice.

It was painful to stand up, sit down or walk. I felt like an old man. Even during our annual retreat in Jamaica, the pain continued, although I had periods of temporary relief from being in the sunshine, from physical movement, and from hot spring soaking. On the way back to the US, I read a book on fasting which inspired me to take on a longer fast with just coconut water. I did not do the fast with the idea that the fast would help my knees. Nonetheless, each day that I continued on the coconut water, my knees felt more and more renewed. I continued for two weeks on the coconut water and, by the end of the fast, the pain in my knees had vanished!

The most interesting part is what came next when I resumed eating my raw food diet. My palate had become very sensitive to salt, so much so that salt felt abrasive to eat. I normally would eat salt-cured olives almost daily, but it took months before I could tolerate once more the salty taste of olives. Through fasting, I had raised my sensitivity to salt to the point where it was undesirable. We need salt just as we need sugar in our food. It is just a matter of the form in which the sugar or salt comes. When sugar is in fresh fruits and vegetables, it is combined with the perfect amount of fiber, water and salt. Salt naturally occurs perfectly in the organic form of sodium in foods, such as celery, green leafy vegetables, and even coconut water. Note a simple daily test to make you aware of when you have eaten too much salt: If you are thirsty after you eat, you have eaten too much salt.

In addition to hypertension, consuming excess amounts of salt creates liquid lime mineral salt deposits to form in the open areas of the joints, causing inflexibility, pain and enlarged joints (e.g., bunions in the feet). Liquid mineral salt is also found in most drinking water. The best way to dissolve these mineral deposits throughout the body is to fast, using fresh distilled water. Coconut water is best, but fresh citrus juice is great too. Fresh orange or grapefruit juice will dissolve the mineral deposits from the joints.

If your diet and habits are not conducive to rejuvenation and health, then disease and illness are inevitable. Some people are naturally ultrasensitive, which is a blessing as their bodies immediately react to poisonous foods. With a destructive lifestyle coupled with being insensitive to daily destruction (i.e., don't get sick or ill often), then what that tells me is that disease is present in your body; it is just not active. The disease is in a latent phase and will erupt sooner or later when it is ready. We all have to recognize where we are and do the best we can. Aspire to improve your diet. Make fasting a part of your lifestyle, and become more sensitive!

FASTING FOR OUR FUTURE

Can we all participate in cleansing through fasting no matter the condition we are in physically? Yes and no. Fasting is the remedy for all disease conditions. All animals in nature undergo a fast when they are injured or feel ill for any reason. When humans fast, the blood immediately thins and that allows for toxins to be eliminated out of the body. When we are injured or scarred, fasting also allows for expedited healing or "speed." The truth is that the body is designed to self-heal. This is why my message is so important, especially when it comes to healing. Despite different doctors, hospitals, healing centers, drugs, herbal supplements, books, journals, the billions spent on research, the billions spent on insurance, and so on, they all come a distant second to scientific fasting done in the way described in this work.

There are certain instances when one has to either prepare him or herself for a fast or do a modified version of the fast. In most instances, a person is either grossly overweight and/or heavily medicated. The level of toxins is too great in the system to even do the liquid portion of the regimen. The most unique case is the instance when there is a new or expectant life involved. I have had a number of women interested in cleansing during their pregnancy or when they are nursing their newborn.

Ideally, a woman and her mate should cleanse, fast, meditate, and do yoga together before the relationship is consummated. By delaying the physical act of sex and directing that sexual energy into your partner through enriching intimate activities, such as fasting, meditation and yoga, you create the best possible scenario for a successful partnership and the creation of a future generation. The art of intimacy should happen through your group meditation and yoga. Sex is the climax of intimacy where you should expect pregnancy and reproduction. Both men and women owe it to themselves to nurture and discipline themselves by creating a serene body temple in which new life is created. We want the best seeds or semen to be planted in the best soil for the best possible child to result. This happens by coming together with the plan of cleansing internally and meditating on the new expectant life you will bring into the world. We are all responsible for our future generation. Fasting in our partnerships is a tool we need to incorporate.

Nonetheless, for the mother who is now pregnant or nursing, is it okay to fast? There is not a straightforward answer. It depends on the diet leading up to conception and birth. The diet leading up to conception is critical, because for most women when they get pregnant, the diet during the pregnancy will largely consist of what the mother is craving. Essentially, the cravings take over. During a pregnancy, the body can be calling for iron, for example. We know that iron is abundant in green leafy vegetables. However, if the mother is used to getting iron from meat or other sources, as opposed to green leafy vegetables, her body will crave that particular food. The body's memory will generate the craving, even at its own expense.

The necessity for a new approach to conception is justified through the understanding of the role of nutrition in the cognitive, physical and spiritual development of the child. The fetus will take what it needs at the expense of the mother. If she plans to have a child, a mother needs to equip herself as far ahead of time as possible. I would say a minimum of two years of preparation for pregnancy is required so that cravings will not dominate her diet at the expense of her body. Women, if you are reading this right now and want or expect to have a child, then imagine a pregnancy free from exhaustion, morning sickness and stretch marks. All three modalities are the result of too much processed cooked starch in the diet. A pregnant woman eating a significant amount of starches during pregnancy will incur excessive weight gain which will lead to morning sickness; exhaustion can result in bed rest. With proper preparation, these issues can be avoided altogether.

The father is not totally off the hook either. For men, it is about our seeds and the quality of our semen. Using fruit as an example think about most of the commercial fruit available today. Seedless fruit is something very common now among fruit that should have seeds, such as watermelon, grapes, and all citrus fruit. Fruit with more seeds has more mineral content and does not spoil as quickly as seedless fruit. I have witnessed seedless watermelon growing fungus in the store! You will never see a heavily seeded watermelon grow fungus even after you buy it and leave it on your counter for a few weeks. Therefore, as men, are we like the excessively hybridized fruit where our seed count is low, or are we like a heavily seeded papaya or watermelon? The quality of our semen has a direct correlation to the quality of our children. Vitality begins with cleansing through fasting to remove obstructions, followed by building our power through exercise and correct food choices.

Women interested in a raw pregnancy should plan for as many years ahead as possible to maintain a raw food diet throughout a pregnancy. When conception happens, a woman should monitor her diet and, as long as there is not any physical or emotional discomfort, she should be able to maintain a raw diet throughout. If a juice regimen is desired, then I would suggest no more than 3 days at a time and that each day's regimen consists of a fresh nut or coconut milk, a vegetable juice and coconut water. With those three components of juices, all nutritional requirements will be met for the woman and her unborn child. Fasting is an art and a science and, when one is on a fast, it needs to be understood that the fast needs to be adjusted at a moment's notice. For anyone pregnant or not, we need to develop the skill of knowing when to break a fast, so that we do not go overboard. It is always better to break the fast and try again soon than to overextend ourselves by fasting too long, only to break the fast incorrectly and overindulge in food.

FASTING AND FEASTING REGIMEN

The question now becomes how do we first undo the mucus that is in every cell and every cell wall lining our bodies? Furthermore, how can we live according to the way in which we were designed to live? The answer to both questions is through proper feasting and fasting.

From my experience and witnessing the experience of others who have fasted unsuccessfully, I have concluded that the best way to fast is to make proper feasting a part of the overall fasting program. What happens too often when we fast, especially when we fast beyond 3 or more days, is that once we take that first bite of food, our cravings take over. In this way, we damage ourselves by overeating the wrong food, and we undo all the sacrifice for the days that we fasted. What is important is that a proper feasting regimen becomes an integral part of the overall plan. The feasting regimen includes a total live food meal or meals that consist only of fresh fruits, vegetables, extra virgin oils and live nut butters, sprouted grains and soaked nuts and seeds.

The next day(s) of our fasting regimen we move into coconut water (or distilled water with fresh lemon or lime) and fresh squeezed orange juice.

Coconut water is Mother Nature's water, as was stated previously. It is naturally distilled water that contains all the vitamins, minerals, and electrolytes the body needs. Between the water and the jelly or meat, we can live and thrive solely on the coconut. Its power comes with the ability to truly nourish you, to allow the body to remove mucus, and simultaneously cleanse all the digestive organs.

NOTE:

For the fast, drink 1 quart of vegetable smoothie for lunch and 1 quart of nut milk for dinner. For the remaining quart of nut milk, I recommend freezing it until the last day of the fast, or sharing with someone else and make more when the time comes for that part of the fasting regimen. Nut milk is very sensitive even in the refrigerator and, in most cases, will spoil after 2-3 days.

After we have completed the OJ/coconut water phase of the fasting regimen, we are then ready to revisit the green smoothie and nut milk. See the Recipe section. We do one day of green smoothies and nut milk, one quart of each drink with coconut water throughout the day. On the final day, we are ready to break fast. The first thing in our mouths is, of course, coconut water, perhaps with a squeeze of fresh lime or lemon juice.

The first solid meal, which is of vital importance, is a mono fruit meal. This meal should be between the hours of 9 AM and 12 PM. The liquids during the fasting regimen have allowed the mucus in the body to become "loose." What that first fruit meal will do is help push the loose mucus out of the body. Some fruits that I would recommend are oranges, grapefruits, grapes, fresh figs, apples, cherries, all berries, papayas, mangos, all melons, pineapples, plums, and pears. Later in the day, sometime between 12 PM and 6 PM, you would prepare your live food feast, but eat minimally to stay in control. If you are hungry after 6 PM, it would be good to drink coconut water or fresh OJ or even another fresh fruit meal.

Khepra's Raw Food Juice Bar 7-Day Detox Regimen

Day	Breakfast	Lunch	Dinner
1	2 lb fresh fruit	Green Leafy Salad with Fresh Fruit (avocado, tomato, papaya, mango, orange); make your own dressing	Repeat lunch
2	32 oz. or more fresh coconut water or fresh citrus juice	32 oz. nut or coconut milk	32 oz. green vegetable juice
3	32 oz. or more fresh coconut water or fresh citrus juice	32 oz. fresh fruit juice (melon or citrus)	32 oz. fresh fruit juice (melon or citrus)
4	32 oz. or more fresh coconut water or fresh citrus juice	32 oz. fresh coconut water	32 oz. fresh coconut water
5	32 oz. or more fresh coconut water or fresh citrus juice	32 oz. fresh fruit juice (melon or citrus)	32 oz. fresh fruit juice (melon or citrus)
6	32 oz. or more fresh coconut water or fresh citrus juice	32 oz. green vegetable juice	32 oz. nut or coconut milk
7	32 oz. or more fresh coconut water or fresh citrus juice	2-3 lbs. fresh fruit (no bananas or dry fruit)	Kale, collard, spinach or romaine green salad with fresh fruit

Khepra's Raw Food Juice Bar 21-Day Detox Regimen

Day	Breakfast	Lunch	Dinner
1	2 lb fresh fruit	Green Leafy Salad with Fresh Fruit	Repeat lunch
2	32 oz. fresh coconut water	32 oz. nut or coconut milk	32 oz. green vegetable juice
3	32 oz. fresh coconut water	32 oz. green vegetable juice	32 oz. green vegetable juice
4	32 oz. fresh coconut water	32 oz. green vegetable juice	32 oz. green vegetable juice
5	32 oz. fresh coconut water	32 oz. fresh fruit juice (melon or citrus)	32 oz. fresh fruit juice (melon or citrus)
6	32 oz. fresh coconut water	32 oz. fresh fruit juice (melon or citrus)	32 oz. fresh fruit juice (melon or citrus)
7	32 oz. fresh coconut water	32 oz. fresh fruit juice (melon or citrus)	32 oz. fresh fruit juice (melon or citrus)
8	32 oz. fresh coconut water	32 oz. fresh coconut water	32 oz. fresh coconut water
9	32 oz. fresh coconut water	32 oz. fresh coconut water	32 oz. fresh coconut water
10	32 oz. fresh coconut water	32 oz. fresh coconut water	32 oz. fresh coconut water
11	32 oz. fresh coconut water	32 oz. fresh coconut water	32 oz. fresh coconut water
12	32 oz. fresh coconut water	32 oz. fresh coconut water	32 oz. fresh coconut water
13	32 oz. fresh coconut water	32 oz. fresh coconut water	32 oz. fresh coconut water
14	32 oz. fresh coconut water	32 oz. fresh coconut water	32 oz. fresh coconut water
15	32 oz. fresh coconut water	32 oz. fresh fruit juice (melon or citrus)	32 oz. fresh fruit juice (melon or citrus)

16	32 oz. fresh coconut water	32 oz. fresh fruit juice (melon or citrus)	32 oz. fresh fruit juice (melon or citrus)
17	32 oz. fresh coconut water	32 oz. fresh fruit juice (melon or citrus)	32 oz. fresh fruit juice (melon or citrus)
18	32 oz. fresh coconut water	32 oz. green vegetable juice	32 oz. green vegetable juice
19	32 oz. fresh coconut water	32 oz. green vegetable juice	32 oz. green vegetable juice
20	32 oz. fresh coconut water	32 oz. green vegetable juice	32 oz. nut or coconut milk
21	32 oz. fresh coconut water	2-3 lbs. fresh fruit (no bananas or dry fruit)	Kale, collard, spinach or romaine green salad with fresh fruits

The above regimens are guides that can be adjusted based on the length of the fast and the specific needs and goals of the individual. For example, if a 21 day fast is done, then the first three days are the same. Instead of doing 'Day 3' for one day in duration, drinking fresh fruit juice can be done for a few days. The coconut water only days should be extended.

The whole idea is that we slowly transition from heavy food, such as dark greens and nuts, to lighter fruits. Beginning the liquid regimen we start with the heaviest juice which is the nut milk. The nut milk is the bridge from fibrous

116

food to liquid juice. In terms of order, the green vegetable juice is the next lightest juice. The fruit juice is next and then we transition to the lightest juice, which is the coconut water. There is a general misconception that green juices detox the body more so than fruit juice and coconut water. Green foods represent building and provide protein and minerals. Foods that provide high nourishment do not detoxify the body. Foods that detoxify are not high nourishers. Fruits are cleansers and will detoxify the body more than greens. Coconut water is lighter than fruit juice and will detoxify the body most optimally while giving the body enough nourishment to allow the faster to have energy during the fast. After a week of coconut water, we reverse the order of juices to prepare the body most optimally to receive food.

SELF-SUFFICIENCY

A successful entrepreneur is one who combines skill, experience, knowledge, heart, and devotion. Above all else, it takes courage. It takes courage to leave a comfy job and follow your passion for life. You leave the security of a regular paycheck, insurance, or a retirement fund.

A good number of people believe 2012 will present an upcoming apocalypse that could take shape in the form of a financial collapse, widespread disease, "terrorist" attacks or some other disaster. One certainty is that December 20, 2012 will end a 26,000-year astrological cycle. It is no coincidence that this major cycle will conclude during the winter solstice. What will actually happen is anyone's guess. Nonetheless, preparing ourselves for some inevitable change is not only wise but also absolutely necessary.

Living in America is living in the land of convenience. However, we pay for these modern conveniences of life. The basic necessities of life are food, water, air, sunlight, and shelter. Beyond that, there is clothing, entertainment, and education, all of which we take for granted. We don't have to farm and harvest our food, fetch our water from the stream, build our houses, or make our clothes. I believe that if we had to do these things daily, we would be much better off, especially from a health perspective. Government and institutions control almost all of our basic necessities. A great disaster could mean that our dependency on food, electricity, gas and water could be snatched right from under us. One approach is to gather bottled water and canned food for the basement. That plan is temporary at best. Something more sustaining would be to secure and own farmland to cultivate and live on and have a fresh water source. By doing so, we reconnect with nature. Our disconnect from nature is the primary reason for all of the world's troubles today, from the individual to the community and to the larger society.

Health insurance is a prime example of creating a lifelong dependency that will allow your health to go through a downward spiral. Paying into a health insurance plan over time, whether it is over years or even decades, will create the idea in your mind that you are taken care of when an eventual health crisis happens. This is the first trap. The second trap is that because you paid into a plan over a significant time period, you would like a return on that investment in your time of need. The idea in your mind is that the particular insurance company should pay for whatever health services that are needed. They OWE you. How can you make a good decision based on your health when you have spent quite possibly a decade paying into a sickcare industry which profits from your ill health? Even for those on Medicaid, the same traps exist even when money earned is not paid out. The options that are paid for are to keep you vaccinated, over-drugged and, perhaps, in line for a surgical procedure.

Now imagine if your insurance plan did not exist. Would that affect how you take care of yourself? Would you eat better? Exercise more? This would be a blessing in disguise. Put the pressure on yourself by taking full responsibility for your health and your life. If you would like to live a long and healthy life, paying into a health insurance plan for 20-30 years that will encourage you to take drugs or go under the knife to cut organs out of you will not guarantee the birthright you have to a long and healthy life. Stop paying for sick care insurance and discover a new lease on life.

The American entrepreneur is someone we can look to as a metaphor for the ideals, such as courage, faith, hope and passion. As Americans, the "New Entrepreneur" of today will have to bring those ideals to another level by sacrificing possibly everything for the sake of survival. What that means is first leaving the US and relocating to a place where business is not put above all else. The ultimate goal is self-sufficiency, and the easiest way to accomplish that is to live in an environment where the temperature is moderately warm year-round. In a warm climate, electricity, gas, heat, and even clothes are not as necessary. One thing is for sure: the urban centers of the world are the cancers of the Earth. Karmically, the cities of the world cannot continue on the path of destruction and consumption of natural resources. The Earth, being the living entity that it is, knows much about detoxifying itself. It has been around much longer and will continue to be around when we are gone. Humans are so egotistical to believe that we can save the Earth. It is up to us to get in harmony with the Earth and Mother Nature, or we will be taken out rather than gracefully pass on. Mother Earth will take out the cities first, because the cities are the tumors and cancers, just as in the human body.

As fasting is Nature's only true healer of the body, I expect the Earth to do nothing short of holding fast and detoxifying. During detoxification, we flush out the garbage through headaches, vomiting, diarrhea, excessive urination, mucus elimination via all parts of the body (skin, ears, eyes, nose, lungs, bowels, urine). Envisioning the Earth as a human body, we can expect volcanoes, hurricanes, earthquakes, tsunamis, tornados and other natural disasters. We should not expect anything less.

We have to work, plan, and pool our resources together to secure livable land in a temperate climate in preparation for the upcoming detoxification of Mother Earth. We need to respect Mother Earth and honor her in everything that we do. When you get into your car, remember that oil has been pumped out of her; basically, every fabric of our lives connects with Mother Earth. Ultimately, we should ask for forgiveness and come into harmony with

Nature's ways for the survival of our species, as we move into an exciting time for us all.

HOW ABOUT SOME FRESH PINEAPPLE FOR DINNER?

If you take anything away from this guide, remember that most of our food must include a high water and moisture content and should primarily come from fresh organic fruits. We are fruitarians. As higher intelligent beings on this planet, we should eat the highest food in its highest form. Most fruits grow up toward the Sun, being pulled up by the Sun's solar rays and energy. That is what we are ingesting, Sun energy, which should be made up mostly of juice and fiber and sometimes seeds. Fruits are the highest vibrational food for the gods of the earth. The higher the fruit grows, elevation-wise, the higher the electric solar energy.

The green water coconut palms grow the highest and have the highest electrical energy contained in the water. This category of nourishment will clean our body, stimulate our mind and nurture our spirit. Grass is for the lower animals, and that includes wheat grass. Cow and goats are in the grass herbivore family of eaters. Grass eaters see green and have the digestive capability to break down tough fibrous grass. Grasses, except for sugar cane, are not fit for human consumption. Our food should include all colors of the rainbow which will insure balance in moisture, vitamins, and minerals.

The fruitarian diet also includes green leafy vegetables, such as lettuces, kale, spinach, collards, turnips, celery, chard, and fresh herbs. It is no coincidence that greens and fruits do not produce any mucus in the body. Those foods should make up 90-100% of our diet. This cannot happen overnight. A regimen of systemic and cyclical fasting, along with doing an occasional fruit day, such as having pineapple for dinner, has to be followed. Pineapple can be substituted with mangos, cherimoyas, berries, peaches, pears, plums, apples, oranges, grapefruits, and melons. This is the ideal diet for longevity and true happiness. The raw diet with today's raw cuisine is a great way to get there. However, too many dehydrated treats and nuts will take its toll on the body. Eating fruits you really enjoy by themselves, along with greens with simple salad dressings, is the ideal diet for the human being.

In our germ conscious society, there is only one way to ensure cleanliness. I can understand why the first raw food movement in the US over 100 years ago was called Natural Hygiene. To put it in perspective, you can sterilize and clean your surroundings, your home and your car; however, your body temple will be filthy and a host for disease because of daily garbage put into the body. Yes, food can be presented well, seasoned and smell great, and even taste great to the palate. Nonetheless, it is nothing but toxic waste in our body temple and has to be managed and stored because the body cannot efficiently assimilate it. We cannot appear to be clean, eat food that turns into pus in the body and then blame a cold, an allergic reaction, sore throat, cough, headache or flu or any other mucus food-derived disease on some external "germ." That germ or virus was created by the dirty food that was consumed. Again, as the saying goes, "You don't catch a cold, you eat one."

True cleanliness comes through the consumption of clean food. Clean food does not produce pus or mucus residue in the body. Clean food includes watermelon, coconuts, sugar cane, jackfruit, apples, and many others. You do not have to worry about using antibacterial soap because, since your diet is clean, it will be naturally equipped and have the intelligence to produce beneficial bacteria and efficiently destroy any harmful bacteria. No sanitizer, plastic gloves, bleach or eating utensils are needed. No colonics, enemas, acidophilus, probiotics, or wheatgrass juice is needed.

RAW CHALLENGE - Eat Living Foods for 100 Days

Eating primarily a raw food diet will slowly detoxify the body. Eating a 100% raw food diet, along with periodic fasting, is what Paradise Health is all about. I've guided hundreds of people on fasts only for them to slowly fall back into their old eating habits. Part of the problem is the lack of know-how. The other part of the problem is that there is not a commitment to stay raw after a week of giving your body well-needed rest and rejuvenation. Given the explosion of popularity in the last 2 decades of the raw food diet, it is reasonable for anyone to commit to doing raw food for at least a 100-day period. The awareness of raw food among health practitioners, celebrities, health enthusiasts and the sick and elderly has allowed the growth of available raw food resources, such as books, DVDs and restaurants for the support needed for success. Many products on the market exist now, that were nonexistent 15 to 20 years ago. For example, there are "Superfoods," coconut water, dehydrated snacks, goji berries, raw food bars, and kombucha, just to name a few. This trend will likely continue.

Over the years, I have seen many people attempt to do a 100% raw food diet and fail. It is not an overnight transition. This is why I am challenging all my readers to commit to doing a 100% raw food diet for at least 100 days. It will take a tremendous amount of will power to overcome cooked food cravings and the peer pressure of social food outings. Time also is not on your side. Each day that goes by is another day on our biological clock. The longer we delay making a change for the better, the more we have to overcome the inevitable challenge of cravings and aging.

Why should anyone do raw or mostly live foods? The short answer is water and enzymes. Our bodies should be at least 70% water. A part of aging is due to our body's percentage of water decreasing over time. It is not enough to drink a lot of water each day. All the food you eat should have some water content. From the mouth to the rectum, what the body is doing is extracting all the water out of the food before it releases the fiber as waste. Therefore, when you eat bread and other starches the body is faced with a monumental task because there is no water drawn out from the fiber and no enzymes to aid digestion. All living foods are equipped with their own digestive enzymes, so that our digestive organs are not excessively taxed with heavy starchy foods that will ultimately clog up our sensitive arteries, organs, and whole body system.

Some research and literature suggests that it takes 21 days to effectively form a new habit. However, twenty-one days is a not a sufficient amount of time to totally transition to a living food diet. On the other hand, if you can do anything for 100 days in a row, then you can do it for the rest of your life. One hundred days encompasses a three-month season, and the number 100 is also psychological. Eating should be looked and treated similarly as with any exercise regimen. In fact, eating is its own internal yoga and is 50% or more of any complete lifestyle improvement program. Eating is the ultimate exercise regimen. Our digestive organs have to work religiously around the clock, extracting, squeezing, moving, and performing miracles for the most part. Out of desperation for rejuvenation, your organs will produce nasal or lung congestion, a headache, virus or skin outbreak, all as signals to tell you to stop eating and give those organs a rest.

What are the main challenges? Cravings and social settings. Cooked food cravings are some of the strongest cravings anyone can face. Cooked starch is at the top of the list. An interesting fact is that whatever the body has the most difficultly with in terms of digesting and processing, the potentially more addictive that food or drug will be. As noted earlier, water and enzymes play a primary role in the food we should eat day in and day out. Cooked starch has no water and no enzymes. How many people are addicted to fruit or vegetables? It's not possible. Even steamed or cooked vegetables are not addictive. Bread is another story. Cooked vegetables may not have enzymes, but they usually have water. We may crave fruits, veggies and water, but an addiction is a false craving that will fulfill something deadly in the body.

Social settings and peer pressure are the other primary hurdles. Cooked food is universally accepted in probably 99% of all social circles worldwide. You can't say the same about cigarettes or even alcohol. At a minimum, it is very important to only involve yourself with vegetarian conscious-minded folk when attempting to make a dietary raw food transition. When I turned raw in 2000, there was not one person I knew with whom I could talk on a daily or even weekly basis for over a year. Now we have raw support groups online, blogs, meet-up groups and potlucks and raw food restaurants. Peer support is critical to success.

For anyone serious about taking on this challenge, please let me know through email, khepra@chefkhepra.com. I will point you to invaluable resources, such as inspirational and informative books, events, markets, retreats, spas, blogs, websites, and so on. Also, please lean on me as your personal support guide. I love to answer questions and will commit myself to seeing everyone succeed. Let's have fun with this.

134

CONCLUSION

Taken from www.dictionary.com, the definition of Paradise is:

• Heaven, as the final abode of the righteous;

• an intermediate place for the departed souls of the righteous awaiting resurrection;

• (often initial capital letter) Eden (def. 1);

• a place of extreme beauty, delight, or happiness; and

• a state of supreme happiness; bliss.

Take this time to congratulate yourself for taking responsibility for your life and your health. Our health is our wealth. We are all our own doctors and self-healers. We can do this better than any health plan, insurance, hospital or holistic health center by proper fasting and feasting. Thank you again for joining the community and me. Having people come together to feast and fast properly gives us the power to effect changes at light speed.

As with any worthwhile journey, it will take work, much determination and focus. Nonetheless, that is the most beautiful part of it —the journey. We must remember each step, especially our breaking points, because they define who we are. Therefore, it is important to journal. Staying consistent with journaling, you will be able to look back to where you were and smile at your daily, weekly, monthly, and yearly progression. Most importantly, we all have the responsibility to help and inspire each other and continue to grow together.

It is important to keep your feasting as light as possible after the fast. Digestion is the Number One energy consumer. Longevity is equivalent to light eating and regular fasting. By doing this fasting and feasting program a number of times throughout the year and the years to come, we come to realize that the body does not receive any energy from food itself. Energy is obtained primarily from oxygen; as we detoxify through proper feasting and fasting—and the addition of a daily morning yoga practice—we will find that our energy shoots up ten-fold during the juice and water period. This increased energy is a result of the higher amount of oxygen contained in the water and juice. This program will not only be a detoxification program but an everyday way of life.

APPENDIX

TESTIMONIALS

Before my spring internal cleansing experience, the longest I'd ever fasted was 1 day, and that was for a medical or physical exam. The first couple of days I experienced slight or minimal headaches twice, but these quickly went away. At no time was I hungry, but it was very hard to be around others when they were eating. Whenever I entered a store, all the snacks seemed to be calling my name and tempting me. However, I stayed strong and persevered, thus experiencing UNBOUNDED PERIODS OF ENERGY. I was constantly moving and felt I needed to do something, so much so that I had to make myself stop and rest. Although I wasn't trying, I lost 6 pounds. Overall, I felt great, lighter and healthier, and I call on everyone to do a quality, weekly fasting or cleansing. Your body, mind and spirit will thank you.

-E. Taylor

This was a wonderful experience that was priceless. To my surprise, I was not hungry during the entire detox. I cooked for my family each day and never was I tempted to taste or eat anything I prepared. This was much easier than I thought. My biggest health improvement was with my sinuses. I have suffered with intense sinus headaches and neck pain for about 10 years. I have tried every prescription and over-the-counter medication and nasal spray, my last being Zyrtec. However, a year ago not even Zyrtec would help, so I started taking apple cider vinegar. This I would do 2 to 3 times a day to keep the headaches away. During this 8-day detox, I have NOT had to take any apple cider vinegar and have had no sinus headaches or neck pain. It feels really good! Good luck. God Bless and you will achieve much success, since this is your passion. THANKS!!

-*C. Lewis*

Blessings from the week: Bills have been paid. Health is great. Energy is up. Stamina is back. Stars are coming into line. God's plan has been manifested. I made it through another week without harm, minimal stress and lots of encouragement.

-*D. Spence*

This has been my first fasting experience. From this experience I have gotten so much; I feel extremely happy and full of energy and less stressed. My cognition has increased and sharpened; my complexion is clearer. My sinus and allergies were suppressed. Intimate moments with my spouse were very beautiful. Initially, I thought absolutely no way I can do an eight-day fasting regimen. I surprised myself and also have learned so much from the members of the group. I have learned how to eat better, breathe better and how to live a healthier and longer life. I WOULD LIKE TO FAST AGAIN WITH THIS GROUP AND ALSO KEEP IN TOUCH WITH EVERYONE.

-R. Rukus

I enjoyed not having to do the work of juicing myself. I usually have to freeze the juice. This way it was prepared fresh daily. I experienced some hunger during the 3 days of OJ, but not much. The key is to consume more water or juice when you feel hunger. I slept very well and had fewer sinus problems. I've been very energized, even though I only slept about 4-6 hours each night. I loved the camaraderie I felt with the group and plan to stay in touch. I also plan to frequent the restaurant when it opens. I've also decided to do my best to convert to a live food diet as I finish the foods I have in my house now. I am highly appreciative of our coordinator, so thankful that God has given me the opportunity to have this wonderful experience.

-S. Tepra

Overall I really enjoyed the fast. I believe that the 1 hour yoga sessions everyday was also a very important and helpful component that should be incorporated into each fast. I did not feel much hunger seeing as this was my first fast. For the past 6-7 months I had been suffering from constant abdominal pain, fatigue and sadness. My body kept telling me it was time to change and this fast was the perfect opportunity for me to take those steps to return back to a healthier lifestyle. My abdominal pain, fatigue and bloating have all dissipated and I have not felt this light, peaceful and energized in almost a year. The spiritual readings and group discussions helped me focus on not only my physical health but my spiritual and emotional health as well. As a 25 year old single woman with no kids I think now is the perfect time for me to continue this journey into holistic wellness. So that when the creator blesses me with a husband and children I can offer them cuisine and a lifestyle enriched by physical activity that my parents were not able to give me. Also being a member of this group has allowed me to meet women 2 and 3 times my senior who offered me support and wisdom and an example to follow. I have never seen so many older women of color who have flawless skin and are in great shape. I can honestly say this fast was a great first step on my personal journey into a healthier lifestyle and a higher consciousness.

-J. Webb

Better sleep. More energy upon arising. Loss of weight. Better body movement and coordination with yoga. Felt great from 1st day of fasting. A joyous experience, a week to remember! Thank you!

-R. Miles

WOW! It has been an amazing week, amazing because I didn't realize how do-able this fast would be; I won't say it was effortless, but it was a lot easier than I expected. When I signed up, I imagined myself being able to stick to the fast for a few days, but not making it the whole way.

I just thought I'd do my best, pay attention to my body and quit if I needed to, but I didn't need to quit. In fact, today is the 8th day of this journey and I could keep going. It was incredibly helpful to be part of this community and to begin each morning with yoga and checking in with one another to see how things were and to wish each other well. The yoga was also a wonderful way to meditate, stretch, and prepare for the day.

Most importantly, it was very helpful to leave here each morning with all the "food" (coconut water & fresh OJ) I needed for the day - and the raw food feast was inspiring. I've spent all week craving that good healthy food, and I look forward to learning how to prepare some of these foods. And, I look forward to the Khepra's Raw Food and Juice Bar opening!!! Thank you for making all this possible.

-M. Tuckey

This fast has opened my eyes to the discipline that I am capable of when I put my mind to it and have a support structure present. When I started the fast, I had a "whatever" attitude, i.e., if I complete this and reach my goal, great; if I don't, that's ok too. But, because of the support of the other participants and the three times we met this past week to discuss our experiences while fasting, I was able to stay focused and reached the end of the fast successfully, not having cheated once (even w/o a piece of gum), which I was tempted to do, but did not do, thankfully. As a result of the fast, and the discipline of which I now know I am capable, I am seriously contemplating taking on a vegetarian lifestyle and attempting to learn live food preparation. The other vegetarian participants in the group have opened my eyes to the vitality of the long-term practice of a vegetarian diet through their youthful appearance, which gives me real inspiration to try vegetarianism in a serious fashion. Overall, this has been an excellent experience and an informative one as well. Through the reading materials provided, I have been educated about the many aspects of my current diet and how it is damaging my health and draining my health and youth. This is definitely something I would do again, given what I have learned and experienced.

-L. Ollie

For me, the fasting has been unique, wonderful and interesting. It has improved or should I say enhanced my ability to be one with All That IS!!

I tend to enjoy large groups of people sharing their experiences. It's more or less a helping tool for me and others. I felt myself becoming more aware of my God, my spiritual being and everyone around me. I especially enjoyed Khepra and all the ladies. The love they displayed was awesome; I fell in love with them. I met so many people on different paths and experiences, WOW!! Love to all of you.

-S. Woods

I must say that this experience has been a true blessing and an experience that I have never had before. I truly feel like a cloud has been lifted from my mind and body. I have been on a natural high and full of energy for this whole week! Doing the Spring Detox with a group made all the difference, keeping me focused and motivated. I have made a connection with each member in the group, which I hope to continue. I have felt a special kind of peace and happiness during the process which is indescribable, making me want to tell everyone with whom I come in contact about it! This experience starts a new chapter in my life, to make different choices about what I consume and maintaining all levels of myself, physically, spiritually, emotionally and mentally. This will also help me to introduce my family to a healthier, more fulfilled lifestyle. I thank everyone involved in this event and all who worked so hard to make it possible.

-K. Whatts

This fast was a wonderful, physically and spiritually enriching experience. The communion with other like-minded folk and the spirit of supportiveness and togetherness was uplifting. The fast itself was well-designed to suit people at all levels. I never felt hungry nor craved food. The early morning yoga helped to wake me naturally and gave me a boost of energy and a positive attitude for the day. This discovery of coconut water as a fasting aid was a "eureka" moment. I'll definitely do this fast again. Please continue or at least repeat it regularly.

-C. Robinson

My personal experience with the fasting of this week was two-fold. The first part was a true test of will to fight temptations all around me. The second part was really the healing process. The yoga really helped with this, uplifting my spirit and helping me get through this week.

-Nico

Just learning about the value of the coconut water for internal cleansing - or shower - as some might say was well worth the cost of the workshop alone. Everything else was a bonus to me; the preparing of the juices for the entire week and the yoga classes, with the option of morning or evening classes, were great also. The raw food was delicious, but most important was the camaraderie and the learning experience with everyone. I Love it and would do it again in a heartbeat!

-Roland

The nut milk was very interesting; I enjoyed it. I also plan to continue this type of fast every other week, because I'm hoping to eventually change my eating habits. I feel that if I continue fasting on a regular basis, I'll continue to slowly eliminate the foods that I shouldn't be eating. This is a fast that one could do regularly. I also enjoyed the yoga classes every morning, though I sometimes struggled. Finally, though I don't overly indulge in things that I should not eat, my ultimate goal is to be as healthy as I can, inside and out. Thank you, Khepra, for the opportunity to once again enjoy your fine cuisine.

-D. Miles

The program was very easy. I never wanted to eat. Now, I feel so light, I am going to do at least 90% live food. Also, I saw an improvement in my body from the first yoga class to the last. This detox will be the beginning of my new body and life.

-J. Ware

I loved this experience. I am really proud of myself for making it through! The live food is delicious!

-M. Lydia

Wonderful cleansing experience. I can't wait to do it again.

-N. Spence

I enjoyed my experience. I was really hungry on Tuesday and Wednesday. The OJ was too thin and not filling enough. I fast, but usually with carrots, spirulina and celery. The 1st meal was awesome! I look forward to the new juice bar opening. The nut milk, WOW! The yoga was good. I practiced, and I enjoyed the level of instruction. On Tuesday, I sat still in bed and felt that I was really in a meditative state. I was communing with God on a level that I never felt before. It was brief, intense and nice. Overall, I enjoyed the fast, especially meeting people who shared it with me. I suggest you do it several times a year, and maybe we can get a group together for other health-related mind-inspiring activities. Thanks for all the effort, work, love and support.

-K. Samara

I followed the regimen exactly as told. I feel great! It was not until Thursday or Friday that I began to feel tired. During the entire process, I did not change the hectic work/home schedule which is why I think I got tired by Friday. During the 8-day regimen, I lost approximately 5 pounds. I had been cleansing myself internally for at least 2 years. I did not get hungry, but I wanted to eat by Thursday, after smelling some good food. One of my co-workers, who did not know about my fast, told me (on Wednesday) that I was glowing! He thought I might be pregnant since I glowed so much. I thanked him and said no! I am just fasting. It has been an awesome experience! The support you provided makes it spiritual, as well as a physical and psychological experience. I truly recommend it to everyone who is interested in improving the quality of their life.

-J. Jackson

This week of fasting and internal cleansing has been a good experience overall. I chose to participate in this program as a part of my journey to perfect health and well-being. My inner voice has been instructing me to get clear. I want to clear my mind, as well as my body, because I have very important life work to do this year. When this opportunity presented itself, I was not sure if I was ready yet, having never fasted before. I nearly chickened out at the last minute, but with a little nudging, decided to go through with it. I am thankful that I did. I learned that live foods are divinely delicious. I also learned that I am more disciplined that I realized. My body did not experience much discomfort. My mind does seem clearer. My ability to focus on work and reading seems better. I regret that my schedule did not permit me to attend the morning yoga classes. I believe yoga would have made a big difference in my experience of the week (for the good). All in all, I feel inspired to leave behind certain poor health choices I'd been making regularly before this week. If I can give up consuming food every day for a week, I can give up unhealthy choices.

-J. May

Dear Khepra,

First, I want to say, 'Thank You,' for hosting the Summer Urban Renewal Detox. I'm still riding high one week after breaking our 6-day juice and water fast. What a remarkably positive experience! I've done two- and three-day fasts in the past, but this was the most effective (and longest) fast I have ever done. I never felt hungry or deprived, nor did any of my usual cravings creep up. In fact, five days into the fast, I went out with friends and was not at all tempted to join them as they shamelessly flaunted their enjoyment of salads, pizza and hot wings). The coconut water you introduced to us is a magical elixir. I was a little concerned that I might have trouble with the two days of only coconut water, but those two days were as easy to get through as the others.

Frankly, I was a little sad that we had to break the fast after 6 days, because I was feeling so good. I could have continued for another week, or more. My energy increased significantly; I required less sleep; I lost several pounds and felt lighter, yet physically stronger. My usual morning mucus cleared up. The early morning yoga helped my flexibility and those annoying mild aches vanished. It was also very helpful to be part of a very supportive and caring group and to come together throughout the week to share our experiences during the fast. Finally, the live food feasts both before and after the fast was absolutely delectable.

Again, thank you for bringing us a safe, sane and satisfying way to fast. This has been the best $250 I've spent all year! I will definitely join you again for another detox session soon.

Peace and blessings, Rene' B.

SHOPPING LISTS

In today's world, which is driven by work, business, family responsibilities, community events and other activities, time becomes everyone's most precious commodity. Taking into account the preparation time for delicious and savory raw and healthy foods, most people are intimidated by these extra time constraints. However, to satisfy the appeal to one's taste buds and recognition of the healthiness of choosing this lifestyle, one has to familiarize oneself with new foods and ingredients, new equipment, sprouting and dehydration. To become the creative genius in your kitchen, it will take time, practice, education and ingenuity. Ultimately, learning to create your food will make your experience more enjoyable, and your body will thank you for your efforts.

It is vital that the new transitions in our kitchens are raised to a higher "kitchen consciousness." We do that by first understanding how and where to get the freshest, healthiest food that we can get. It may mean driving an extra few miles to the market that sells organic produce. You will have to familiarize yourself with local farmers' markets, especially for your green leafy vegetables. You will need to dust off your juicers, food processors and dehydrators. Your dehydrator should replace your microwave and stove. In addition, having a good set of knives with a high-powered blender should fulfill your kitchen needs.

For raw food cuisine, there are dishes that are repeated more often than not. Those would include nut pâtés, greens, sprouted grain salads, vegetable fruit salads, dressings, sauces and desserts. Over the years, I continually have made variations of these dishes and have learned that there is a commonality present. By this I mean that I don't necessarily incorporate the same ingredients but the *same category* of ingredients. For example, garlic, onions, leeks, scallions, ginger and shallots all belong to the mustard family, so they can be used interchangeably for the most part.

In the following section, we will look at the key categories/families of foods that form the key cornerstones of most living recipes. Those "families" are the following: mustard, sour, hot, fresh herb, dried spice, salt, oil and sweet. The lists below are not exhaustive but include the most commonly used foods. Also included are common ingredients which always should be part of your kitchen foodstuffs.

Mustard Family

Onion

Garlic

Scallion

Leeks

Chives

Ginger

Shallots

Sour Family

Lemon

Lime

Sour orange

Apple cider vinegar

Red wine vinegar

Balsamic vinegar

Hot Family

Jalapeño pepper

Scotch Bonnet/Habanero peppers

Cayenne pepper

Chile pepper

Fresh Herb Family

Thyme

Rosemary

Sage

Basil

Oregano

Cilantro

Parsley

Dill

Marjoram

Tarragon

Bay leaves

Mint

Chervil

Dried Spice Family

Allspice

Celery seed

Cinnamon

Curry

Cumin

Nutmeg

Salt Family

Celtic sea salt

Himalayan sea salt

Nama Shoyu

Miso

Black salt

Real salt

Sea vegetables

Oil Family

Olive oil

Coconut oil

Palm oil

Sesame oil

Tahini

Sweetener Family

Coconut nectar

Dates

Raisins

<u>Fresh</u>:

Avocado

Tomato

Plantain

Collards

Kale

Spinach

Mustard greens

Celery

Zucchini (soft)

Bell peppers (red, orange, yellow)

Lemons

Limes

Cucumbers

Mushrooms (Portobello, Shitake)

Seasonal Fresh Fruit:

Peaches

Apples

Mangos

Oranges

Berries

Pineapple

Raw Nuts & Seeds:

Pecans

Almonds

Cashews

Pine nuts

Walnuts

Sunflower seeds

Pumpkin seeds

Flax seeds

Pistachios

Condiments:

Vanilla extract

Apple cider vinegar

Red wine vinegar

Extra virgin olive oil

Nut Butters:

Almond

Hemp

Tahini

Dried Fruit:

Medjool dates

Raisins

Sundried tomatoes

Olives

Cacao

Maca

Grains:

Quinoa

Garbanzo beans

Buckwheat groats

Wild rice

Frozen:

Corn

Peas

Sea Vegetables:

Wakame

Dulse

Hijiki

Arame

Kelp

Nori

Equipment List:

Quality knives & cutting board

Cuisinart food processor

Vitamix blender

Citrus juicer

Excalibur dehydrator

Champion juicer

RECIPES

Whether it is a nut pâté, a salad or a dressing, the categories above form the foundation for creating delectable, tasty recipes. Below are examples of some foods that can be combined to put together quick dishes.

Nut Pâté:

A nut pâté is a nice way to get an abundance of protein and healthy fat. Soak all your nuts and seeds for at least 8 hours, drain and rinse thoroughly. Keep them refrigerated or frozen if not using right away.

2 cups nuts/seeds of your choice, soaked 8 – 12 hours

¼ cup fresh vegetables (celery, beets, carrots, tomato, etc.)

¼ cup ingredient from the Mustard family

1 Tbs. ingredient from the Hot family

1 Tbs. – ¼ cup from Herb family

1 Tbs. dried ingredient from Dried Spice family

1 Tbs. from Salt family

Grind the nuts/seeds in a food processor and add the remaining ingredients to the ground nuts in a mixing bowl. Enjoy as a spread or form into patties and dehydrate.

Green Salad & Dressings:

Eating green leafy vegetables is absolutely critical for good health, especially if you live in a colder climate. Therefore, it is imperative to be creative with your greens, so that it is never boring. All your fruits, sweet and non-sweet, can be combined with your greens with the exception of melon fruits. Adding soaked seeds, such as pumpkin, hemp or sunflower, wonderfully complements any green salad.

1 head of greens of your choice

1 cup fresh vegetables and/or fruit

½ cup soaked seeds

Dressings & Sauces:

½ cup olive oil

¼ cup ingredient from Mustard family

1 Tbs. ingredient from Hot family

1 Tbs. ingredient from Sour family

1 Tbs. – ¼ cup from Fresh Herb family

1 Tbs. ingredient from Dried Spice family

1 Tbs. ingredient from Salt family

Add all ingredients to bowl and mix well.

Sprouted Grain Salad:

Sprouting is a process that takes at least 24 – 36 hours, depending upon the grain. Quinoa is great because it is alkaline forming and only takes 12 hours to sprout. Most grains will take longer to sprout after soaking.

1 cup Sprouted Grain

½ cup fresh vegetables (celery, beets, carrots, tomato, etc.)

¼ cup ingredient from Oil family

¼ cup ingredient from Hot family

1 Tbs – ¼ cup ingredient from Fresh Herb family

1 Tbs. ingredient from Sour family

1 Tbs. ingredient from Dried Spice family

1 Tbs. ingredient from Salt family

Add all ingredients to bowl and mix well.

Vegetable Fruit Salad:

Vegetable fruits are fruits that have little or no sugar. This is another area of any raw menu in which your creativity can soar, since there are so many foods from which to choose. What I use most commonly are avocados, tomatoes, peas, corn, olives, pumpkin, zucchini, currants, bell peppers and plantains.

2–3 cups chopped vegetable fruits

¼ cup ingredient from Oil family (optional)

¼ cup ingredient from Mustard family

1 Tbs. ingredient from Hot family

1 Tbs. – ¼ cup from Fresh Herb family

1 Tbs. ingredient from Sour family

1 Tbs. ingredient from Dried Spice family

1 Tbs. ingredient from Salt family

Add all ingredients to bowl and mix well.

Dessert:

This is a quick way to create a sweet dessert without too much prep time.

1 cup soaked nuts

2–4 cups fresh seasonal fruit

½ cup from Sweetener family

1 tsp. vanilla extract

1 Tbs. from Dried Spice family (usually cinnamon or nutmeg)

Dash of sea salt

Grind nuts in food processor with spice, sweetener, salt and vanilla extract. Pulse fruit, sweetener and vanilla extract (optional with the fruit or nut mixtures). Coconut oil also can be used with the fruit. Lay out the nut mixture in a dish with fruit on top and serve.

Listed below are some examples of actual recipes that follow the formula for creating a recipe above. These are great recipes to introduce into your dietary routine following a fasting regimen. The key with live food preparation is simplicity. Of course, as Mother Nature is the ultimate chef, coming off a juice fast, especially an extended one, your body will only want one food at a time. Therefore, it is highly recommended that your first meal or your first few meals be a mono diet of primarily fruits. By eating mono, you would just eat watermelon with seeds, for example. Chew the watermelon seeds with the flesh. They are very tasty and are a great source of protein. Any fruit would be great, such as cucumbers, figs, tomatoes, strawberries, mangos or sweet bell peppers. After a fast, your taste buds are sensitive and become acquainted with Mother Nature as the one and only true chef of food creation. Mixing foods with spices, herbs, sugar and salt allows us to first overeat, second, over stimulate our palate, and third, not taste food for truly how it is meant to taste. Recognize and compartmentalize your proteins, fats, sweets, starches, herbs, spices and so forth when creating. Remember that less is more.

Savory Avocado-Plantain Pie:

Avocado

Medjool dates

Plantain

Celery

Spinach

Red bell pepper

2 cups cashews

Fresh herbs

½ sundried tomatoes

Onion

Apple cider vinegar

Nut Meat Crust (see below)

Red wine vinegar

Savory Tomato Binder (see below)

Garlic

Cashew Pine Nut Cheese (see below)

Spread nut meat crust evenly throughout bottom of dish. Assemble plantains. Spread cheese evenly over plantains. Add layer of chopped spinach. Spread cheese or tomato paste over spinach. Assemble avocado. Spread cheese or tomato paste over avocado. Allow to set in refrigerator for a few hours to gel or serve immediately.

Nut Meat:

3 cups walnuts, almonds or pecans, soaked overnight

2 cups celery, chopped

½ medium onion, chopped

1 clove garlic

¼ cup parsley, chopped

¼ cup red pepper, chopped

1 Tbs. olive oil

1 Tbs. sea salt

Thoroughly rinse nuts and then process in a food processor or homogenize in a Champion juicer with blank plate. Place ground nuts in a bowl, add remaining ingredients and mix well.

Savory Tomato Paste:

3 medium Heirloom tomatoes

1 cup sundried tomatoes

½ cup dates

½ cup red bell pepper, chopped

1 celery stalk, chopped

Few fresh sprigs of fresh rosemary and/or parsley

1 tsp. Italian seasoning

Combine all ingredients except fresh tomatoes in a food processor with S-blade and process for a few minutes. Add fresh tomatoes until you have desired consistency.

Cashew Pine Nut Cheese:

2 cups cashews, not soaked

2 cups pine nuts, not soaked

1 cup apple cider vinegar

¼ cup Nama Shoyu

1 cup coconut water

Grind nuts with S-blade and process for a few minutes. Add remaining ingredients for desired consistency.

Curried Wild Rice:

2 cups wild rice, soaked

¼ cup parsley, chopped

¼ cup scallions, chopped

1 tsp. Indian curry powder

1 Tbs. almond butter

1 tsp. black salt, real salt or Nama Shoyu

½ cup Extra Virgin olive oil

¼ cup red wine vinegar

1 Tbs. basil or thyme, chopped

Soak wild rice for 24 hours, rinsing and changing the water at 8-hour intervals. Combine all ingredients together. Mix well and enjoy.

<u>Sea Relish</u>:

2 cups Wakame

1 cup Dulse

Couple of sheets of Nori

¼ cup parsley, chopped

¼ cup scallions, chopped

¼ bell pepper, chopped

¼ cup tomatoes, chopped

1 Tbs. basil or thyme, chopped

Soak sea vegetables for 15 minutes in coconut water. Combine all ingredients together. Mix well and enjoy.

Fresh Greens:

4 cups fresh greens of choice (kale, collards, spinach)

1 cup Extra Virgin olive oil

1 Tbs. black salt

¼ cup red wine vinegar

¼ cup bell pepper, chopped

¼ cup garlic and/or onions, diced

1 Tbs. coconut nectar

Combine all ingredients together. Mix well and enjoy.

Chocolate Nut Milk:

3 cups soaked almonds or Brazil nuts

6 cups water

4 bananas

7 dates

1 tbs. cacao nibs

1 cup Extra Virgin coconut oil

½ tsp. vanilla

½ tsp. Celtic sea salt

Combine all ingredients in a blender. Blend thoroughly and strain. Yields ½ gallon of nut milk.

Berry Cream Pie:

(This is a quick way to create a sweet dessert without too much prep time.)

2 cups nuts (pecans or walnuts), soaked overnight

2–4 cups fresh seasonal fruit

½ cup coconut nectar

1 tsp. vanilla extract

Dash of sea salt

Cashew Cream (see below)

Grind nuts in a food processor with spice, sweetener, salt and vanilla. Pulse fruit with dry fruit, sweetener and vanilla. The vanilla is optional with the fruit or nut mixtures. Coconut oil also can be used with fruit. Lay out the nut mixture in a dish with the fruit on top and serve.

Cashew Cream:

2 cups cashews, not soaked

½ cup fresh lemon or lime juice

¼ coconut nectar

½ tsp. vanilla

½ cup coconut oil

Dash of sea salt

Grind nuts in a food processor. Add the remaining ingredients and continue to process. Add as the layer in the dessert dish with fruit on top and serve.

There are many live food recipes that can be found via the internet and books that have been published in the last 5 years to help guide you on your way to becoming a live food chef in your very own kitchen.

After doing at least one day of live foods or a proper feasting regimen, we then move into the fasting regimen. The first day consists of fresh coconut water for breakfast, nut milk for lunch and vegetable green juice for dinner, with coconut water in-between, if thirsty throughout the day. If coconut water is not available, the next best thing is distilled water or reverse osmosis water with fresh lemon juice or lime juice added to it.

Here are a couple of sample recipes for the vegetable smoothie and a nutmilk:

<u>Green High Juice</u>:

1 bunch of kale or collards

4 cups of coconut water

1 cup of apple, pear or pineapple

Small piece of ginger (optional)

Combine all ingredients in a blender and blend thoroughly. Milk the juice through a nut milk bag or cheesecloth. Yields 2 quarts of green juice.

Coconut Milk:

1 cup tender coconut meat or jelly

5–6 cups coconut water

Blend thoroughly and strain, if necessary. Yields ½ gallon of coconut milk.

BIBLIOGRAPHY

Ehret, Arnold, Mucusless Diet Healing System, New York, NY, Benedict Lust Publications, 2002.

Ehret, Arnold, Rational Fasting, New York, NY, Benedict Lust Publications, 2002.

Fife, Bruce, Coconut Water: For Health and Healing, Colorado Springs, CO, Piccadilly Books, Ltd., 2008.

Hotema, Hilton, Man's Higher Consciousness, Pomeroy, WA, Health Research Books, 1962.

Shelton, Herbert M., Fasting Can Save Your Life, Tampa, FL, American Natural Hygiene Society, Inc., 1978.

CPSIA information can be obtained
at www.ICGtesting.com
Printed in the USA
BVHW042025250420
578480BV00009B/1273